WHAT TO DO

UNTIL THE

VET ARRIVES

Emergency Care for Horses

NANCY S. LOVING, DVM

Author of *All Horse Systems Go* and *Go the Distance*

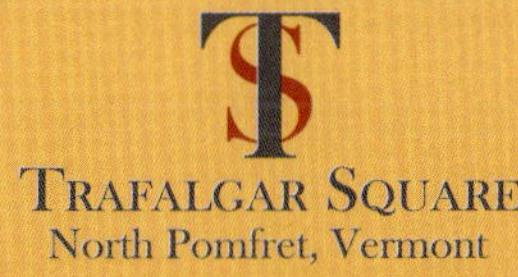

TRAFALGAR SQUARE
North Pomfret, Vermont

First published in 2025 by
Trafalgar Square Books
North Pomfret, Vermont 05053

Library of Congress Cataloging-in-Publication Data is available on file.

Photographs courtesy of Nancy S. Loving except: pp. 10, 14, 15, 24, 27, 32, 34, 80, 127 right, 133 (by Abigail Boatwright), pp. 1, 42 bottom left/right, 43 top right, 163 (Adobe Stock), and p. 150 (by Ray Randall, DVM)

Book design by Lauryl Eddlemon
Index by Andrea Jones (JonesLiteraryServices.com)
Cover design by RM Didier

Printed in China

10 9 8 7 6 5 4 3 2 1

This book is dedicated to all my equine patients and their owners who diligently care for them as family members, doing the best for their horses as possible. No emergency is ever the same and timely actions and calls for veterinary assistance yield the best outcomes. The horses have taught me so much over the span of many decades, not just about nuances of veterinary medicine but also for their depth of partnership with their human caretakers. Despite the pain, discomfort, and fear the horses may feel in the throes of a crisis, their trust in us who come to their aid is simply inspirational.

CONTENTS

Part 3: Preparing for General Emergencies 153

Alphabetical Quick Reference of
POSSIBLE EMERGENCIES

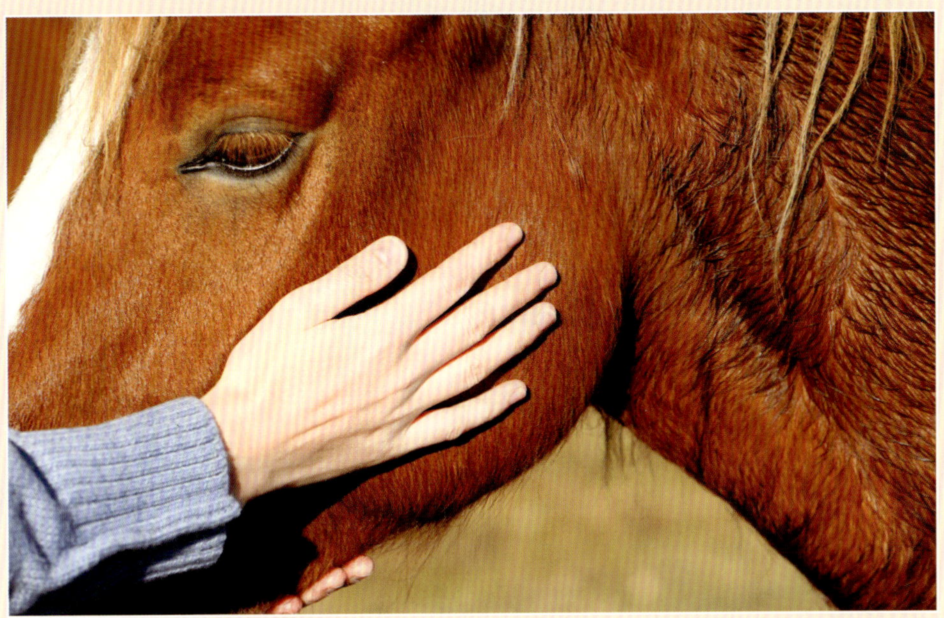

INTRODUCTION

As a responsible horse owner, you always want to do what's best for your horse. So what do you do when you're faced with an emergency crisis but professional veterinary health care is difficult to access? In the short term while awaiting professional veterinary help for an emergency, there are specific strategies you can use to help your horse, while also improving the outcome of the problem.

This book will explore many common emergencies that horse owners face. It's important to know what exactly constitutes an emergency and also what steps you can take to help your horse through it.

There are many ways to achieve the same results but only if you have some way to evaluate the problem you're facing, and some idea where to start. Here in these pages are tools and assessments you can use and options you can try. At all times, it is critical that you stay safe. If a horse doesn't want to be handled during his crisis, then the best choice is to wait for the veterinarian to arrive or put the horse in a trailer and haul him to a professional veterinary facility. Horses can be volatile and unpredictable, especially when experiencing pain. Please take care!

PART 1

EQUINE
EMERGENCY
BASICS

WHAT CONSTITUTES AN EQUINE EMERGENCY?

There are many situations that cause panic in a horse owner, and while they are upsetting, not all of them are *true emergencies*.

It is important to evaluate the whole horse and not just focus solely on an obvious concern. It is common for more than one problem to have occurred that needs immediate attention. While you focus on a gaping wound on your horse's leg, you might fail to notice another laceration along the abdomen or elsewhere. Or, the wound you are dealing with turns out to have occurred during a mild colic crisis that caused the horse to roll into a fence.

A thorough inspection of all sides and parts of the horse will help you identify all the issues you need to address, not just the most obvious one.

WHAT ARE EXAMPLES OF TRUE EMERGENCIES?

A *true emergency* is one that threatens a horse's life or physical health and needs to be resolved as soon as possible.

In no particular order, and certainly not exhaustive of all possibilities, here are some examples of emergencies that are helped by immediate action:

- Lack of appetite.

- Fever.

- Intestinal issues: colic; choke; abnormal manure (diarrhea, or dry, hard fecal balls).

- Eye trauma.

- Respiratory illness or duress.

- Acute onset significant lameness—laminitis; hoof nail puncture; hoof abscess; fracture.

- Acute musculoskeletal swelling, especially if associated with joints or tendons.

- Wounds, including hemorrhage, lacerations, or injuries to synovial structures like joints or tendons.

- Snakebite.

- Poisoning.

- Neurological problems—incoordination (ataxia), physical weakness, or changes in cognition or mental status.

Not only is it important to deal with the immediate problem, but it is also essential to ensure no further harm comes to a horse during or after an injury or illness. Don't ride a horse with a swollen tendon; have lameness evaluated as timely as possible; administer care for a painful eye; tend to a wound or laceration; don't ignore a horse's waning appetite; and always check rectal temperature if the horse isn't acting right or is off his feed.

MEDICAL CONSENT AND INSURANCE CONSIDERATIONS

In advance of a crisis, it is worth engaging in some thought exercises to decide how far you'd be willing to go to resolve your horse's problem. You'll want to have a game plan once your veterinarian arrives, especially if the horse must be transported to a referral facility. In some emergencies, every minute matters, so it is best to have thought this through beforehand, ideally during a calm, non-emergency period.

Consider:

- Cost of emergency care and follow-up procedures, including surgery.

- Potential for continued athletic use.

- Difficulty or ease of care and rehabilitation, how long that might take, and if you have the facilities to accomplish this.

- Whether or not the horse is insured for medical problems, and/or loss of use.

Once you decide to go forward with managing a crisis, assign a specific dollar value to how much you are willing to invest in your horse's emergency care. Keep in mind that colic surgery now runs at least $5,000, and follow-up needs add to this amount.

Prepare a document stating your exact wishes regarding what can be done for your horse. Include:

- The highest dollar value you'll invest and your decisions to consider if care exceeds this amount.

- How to handle a situation where the horse has no potential for future athletic use.

- Instructions for consent to euthanasia if that is the most humane option as evaluated by a veterinary professional.

- Instructions for obtaining a second opinion if you do not want the horse euthanized in your absence or until another veterinarian concurs that euthanasia is the most humane option.

If the horse is insured, have all insurance information at hand.

- Post equine insurance information and contacts on the stall and/or in an office and inform others where it can be found.

- Provide this information to your veterinarian and to your proxy person prior to an emergency.

- It is necessary to obtain permission from an equine insurance agency for many procedures before they can be performed by veterinary professionals.

If you are not present or available at the time of an equine emergency crisis, provide a list of veterinarians to call if you are not available. Have contact information for a designated person (proxy) or persons who have agreed in advance to "speak" for you and make decisions on your behalf if you cannot be reached. And provide them with your credit card information to expedite care. Include information about allergies a horse may have, including to medication, and if there are dietary specifications.

Update all this information annually as your circumstances and desires may change.

SAFETY CONSIDERATIONS

SAFE PLACE TO TREAT

When tending to your horse's emergency, begin by assessing the problem. Ensure that you have a safe environment to work on your horse, in an area free of obstacles and equipment. Survey the surroundings and consider potential hazards that thwart safety.

- If working outside, avoid areas with large machinery—tractors, horse trailers, pickup trucks and cars, and mowing equipment, for example.

- When working inside, keep barn aisleways clear of obstacles—rakes, manure forks, wheelbarrows, saddles, tack, equipment, and chairs. Store this equipment in appropriate places to avoid finding it in your or your horse's way in an emergency.

- Look carefully at all edges and corners of walls and stalls. Check for chewed or broken pieces of wood, splinters, nails, or bolts protruding from posts or boards.

- Ensure that aisle mats fit snugly to each other and flat on the floor to avoid a horse or person tripping on an uneven edge.

- Check ceiling height and light fixtures that pose a hazard to a rearing horse that could smash his head on an unprotected fixture or metal beams.

- Remove electrical cords that pose a hazard while tending to the horse, especially if working in a wet area.

- Make sure that horses, people, children, and small animals (dogs, cats, chickens, ducks, geese) are out of the way and not likely to wander back into your work area. This is really important to prevent other accidents from occurring.

Not every horse stands quietly for medical ministrations, so carefully evaluate the treatment area to prevent the possibility of further injury if a horse explodes violently. It is equally as important to protect yourself and assistants by ensuring there is ample space to move out of harm's way.

Once you have identified a clear space free of hazards and obstacles, you can begin to tend to your horse.

SAFE RESTRAINT

Working on a horse with an emergency crisis requires a cool head and attention to detail. It is safe to proceed with emergency first aid *only* if the horse is cooperative and allows treatment. If the horse is fractious and unruly, do not proceed; wait for professional help.

Efficient handling of a horse relies on effective control and decisive actions by the handler. Confidence in your actions reassures a horse he can trust in you.

Horse Control

Proper restraint of the horse is paramount for safety.

- This starts with a halter and lead rope that are in good working condition. Always halter a horse for control before administering any medical care or procedure. Do not try to control a horse by directly holding onto his halter. Do not lead a horse by holding on to his halter—use a strong lead rope securely affixed to the halter ring.

  - The halter should fit well—not too tight and not too loose.

  - A soft lead rope is less abrasive to your hands and provides the best control. For handling a difficult horse, it helps to wear gloves.

  - Don't wrap a lead rope around your hand and take care with rope handling when wearing jewelry.

  - Check that the snap on the end of the rope is strong and secures properly when closed.

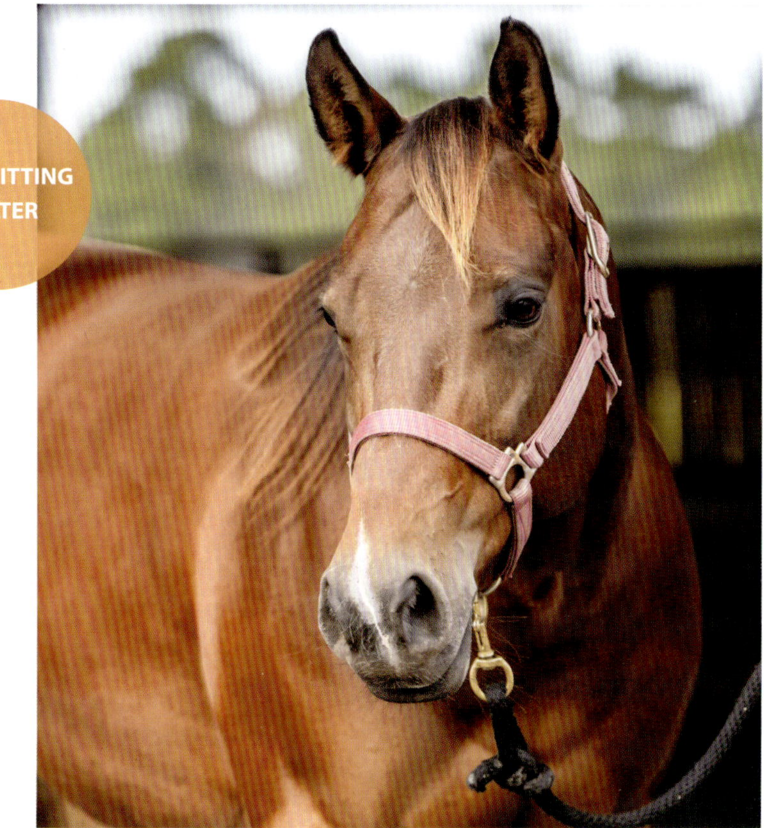

A halter that fits well.

- If a halter is not available, a soft rope can be turned into a halter. Form a loop of rope around the horse's neck and secure it with a bowline knot that won't jam when tightened. Then, pass another loop of rope through the neck loop and over the nose to form the face part of a halter. The remaining length of rope serves as a "lead rope."

- Lead using two hands on the rope—one hand near the horse's head (not too tightly and not too loosely) with the other hand holding the long end of the rope off the ground.

- When possible, have a capable assistant handle and hold the horse while you examine and minister to the horse.

- Wear appropriate closed-toe footwear. Do not work around horses wearing sandals!

- For all persons ministering to the horse, avoid distractions—don't talk on a cell phone or to others milling about in the barn. Keep your attention focused on the horse and the task at hand at all times, and your senses tuned to all goings-on around you.

- It is best to discourage hand feeding of treats, as horses may not pay attention or may become pushy and aggressive about getting treats.

- Never tie or cross-tie a horse to anything—solid or loose—for a procedure that involves possible pain or discomfort to the horse in case he becomes reactive.

  - If the horse is tied securely and pulls back, pulling an object away from a wall or fence and it remains attached to the lead rope, the horse will be terrified by this flailing post, fence piece, or other object. This poses a serious hazard to both the horse and any humans around him.

  - If you are using cross-ties for grooming or inspection, attach the end snaps to breakable cord—baling twine, for example. If the horse tries to rear up in the cross-ties, the twine will break and release him rather than causing him to flip over backward, which could ultimately cause a life-threatening injury.

- • If a horse doesn't tie well, then loop his lead rope around something without tying it; this way, if he pulls back, the rope will loosen and he won't feel trapped by pressure.

- • Have a knife handy in your pocket or clipped to your belt for immediate access so you can cut a rope if needed to free an entangled horse.

- ■ If a horse is anxious about being alone while being treated, the presence of a horse buddy in a nearby paddock or stall can be calming.

- ■ A horse bothered by flies may not stand quietly for work on his legs. Use fly spray or run a fan to deter flies from landing.

Safe Positions for Handler and Examiner

- ■ Never stand directly in front of the horse; handle him from the side. If you are in front of a bolting or spooking horse, it is difficult to get out of the way in time. Standing to the side within a safety zone (within 1½ feet or less) gives you the best control of his head and body.

- ■ The handler stands facing forward, to the side of the horse's head and shoulder, with a firm grip on the lead rope, holding it about 3 feet from the snap. Too much rope length enables a horse to move in too many directions, which is dangerous; too tight a hold restricts the horse's head, which can cause him to feel pressured enough to elicit a reaction.

- ■ Don't let a horse run past a handler; this puts other people in danger of a swift, targeted kick.

- ■ Positions for a handler to stand while the examiner is tending to the horse:

- On the opposite side of the horse, when the examiner works on a front limb.

- On the same side, when the examiner is working on the horse's back end. If the horse threatens or menaces the examiner, the handler can turn the horse's head towards both people to swing the horse's butt away, which will keep both examiner and handler out of range of a kick.

- Out of range of the swing arc of any leg or the horse's neck for an injured or sick horse lying on the ground. It is preferable to work from *behind* the prone horse's back, up by the withers, and reach across his body as necessary.

Restraint Devices

Use all restraint devices and techniques with caution, as any horse may explode violently when restrained, without any forewarning. Use these devices with kindness and respect for the horse. Used incorrectly, a restraint device could be abusive and cause a horse to react violently, which is the opposite of what you are trying to accomplish.

Familiarize yourself with how to use restraint devices safely and know what restraints your horse accepts or doesn't accept. If a horse doesn't respond favorably to restraint tactics, It Is besl lo forgo attempts at treatment and instead rely on a veterinary professional as soon as possible to avoid injury to horse or handler.

Possible restraint devices:

- A *twitch* is applied to the upper nose. This can be a metal or wooden twitch, or a loop of baling twine twisted taut over the end of the nose.

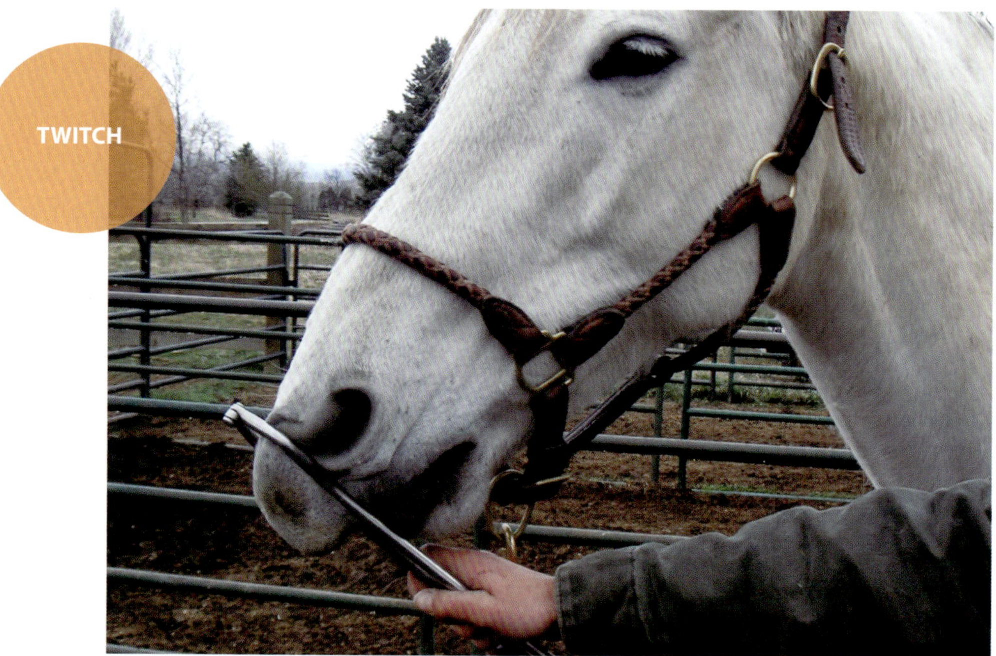

A twitch correctly applied.

The shank of an applied solid twitch is held relatively perpendicular to the horse's nose and the ground without twisting the nose.

- A *lip chain* is an excellent restraint tool when used properly. If no chain is available, substitute a piece of rope or strong baling twine. The beauty of a lip chain for those horses that tolerate it is that the horse is rewarded automatically when he behaves well. The chain is placed beneath the upper lip and over the upper gum line to exert pressure when a horse doesn't yield to ministrations. If he struggles by lifting his head or trying to turn or escape, he feels increased pressure on his gums from the lip chain. As soon as he stops the behavior, he is rewarded with instant relief. Maintain just enough tension to keep the

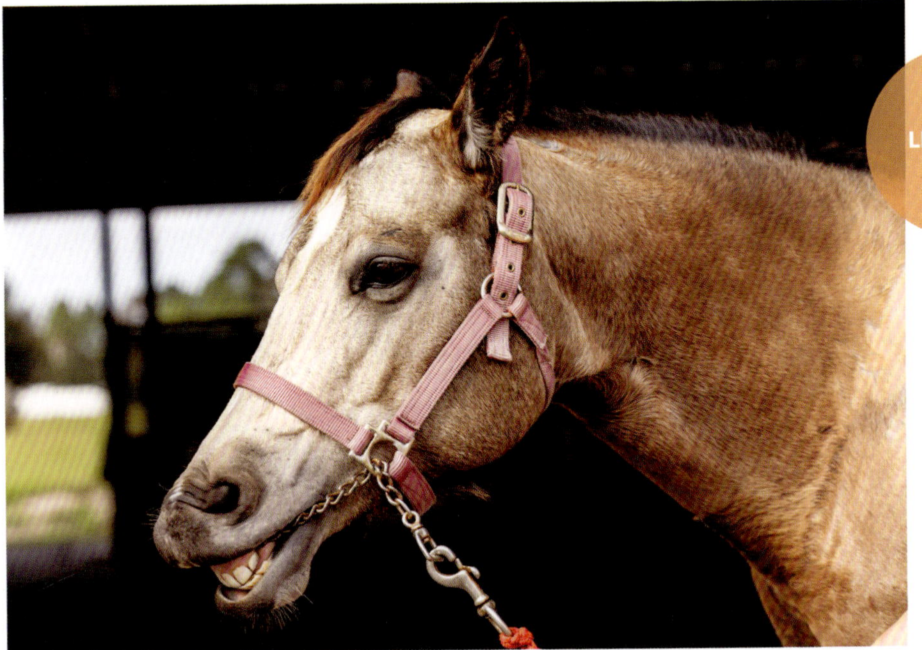

A lip chain in place as a means of restraint during emergency care.

chain situated in place on the gums so it doesn't loosen and fall off. Tension can be increased if the horse behaves badly.

- A *skin pinch* works well on some horses. Grab and squeeze a large wad of neck skin in your hand.

- An *ear hold* may work for some horses but should be used judiciously as this restraint can amplify adverse behavior, especially in horses that are ear shy. Pull the ear down gently without twisting and hold firmly.

- A *blindfold* over both eyes is helpful to calm a horse enough for him to stand quietly. Any cloth material is usable as long as it completely covers both eyes and won't slip loose.

FIRST AID KIT

Preparation for an emergency helps you keep a level frame of mind and gives you confidence you can deal with a calamity. You may have everything ready at hand for a horse emergency yet never need to dive into the first aid kit. While ideal, this is probably unlikely, since horses are inquisitive and energetic, and just about anything can happen. Robert Baden-Powell, founder of the Boy Scouts, proclaimed, "A Scout is never taken by surprise; he knows exactly what to do when anything unexpected happens." Such a sound approach is appropriate to stocking a first aid kit that arms you with options, plus the knowledge of what to do.

Many supplies for a first aid kit are available over-the-counter or from a veterinarian, while some medications need a veterinarian's prescription and guidance. Be sure you understand how to use prescription medications and use them only under advisement from your veterinarian.

You'll want your stocked first aid kit—containing materials and supplies—to be easily accessible. However, it is important to store all first aid supplies and medications out of reach of young children, pets, and other people you don't want accessing them, under lock and key if necessary. Keep everything dust-free and dry, and at a constant temperature, neither too hot nor too cold. Store drugs at the manufacturer's recommended temperature to prevent loss of the drug's efficacy. Check expiration dates on medications and supplies once or twice a year; replace and update as needed. Dispose of medications responsibly—contact a veterinarian for this purpose.

Storage Container

Ideally, all your first aid supplies are stored in a clean, dry environment. A plastic storage container works well for this purpose. When supplies are emptied from the container, it can serve as a basin to hold water so you can make a physiologic salt solution (saline) for cleansing a wound or irrigating an eye.

- Fill the container with a quart of water and mark a line on the outside with indelible ink or tape for future reference.

- Prepare multiple pre-measured baggies with ½ tablespoon of table salt in each.

- To make a saline solution, dissolve ½ tablespoon of salt in one quart of water—which you can now do by filling your container with water up to the line you marked, and then emptying one of your baggies into it, stirring until it is well dissolved.

- Refer to the section on wound care (starting on p. 97) for details on how to use supplies.

Items to Include in the First Aid Kit

Contact Information

- A card or laminated paper that includes phone numbers for your veterinarian, an emergency veterinary hospital, and a farrier. Also include your own phone contact information and that of a friend who is willing to act as proxy agent on your behalf in your absence.

Supply List

- A list of everything contained in your first aid kit so you can ensure that supplies you've used (which should be crossed off once removed) will be replaced. Adding expiration dates helps you keep your supplies up-to-date.

Restraint Tools

- For example, a twitch, lip chain, or blindfold material.

Wound Cleansing Materials

There is a saying that "cleanliness is next to godliness," and this applies when it comes to wound care—cleanliness is the best way to deter infection. To most effectively clean a wound, you'll want to have the following on hand:

- Disposable razor or scissors to remove hair around a wound.

- Gauze sponges (3 inches x 3 inches) for scrubbing. Only use cotton for scrubbing if you can ensure no fibers are left in a wound. Soak gauze or cotton in saline solution before scrubbing a wound.

- Antiseptic (povidone-iodine or chlorhexidine) solution to add to saline for rinsing and irrigating wounds. Use 10 milliliters of povidone-iodine or 20 milliliters of chlorhexidine per liter (or quart) of salt water.

- Antiseptic (povidone-iodine or chlorhexidine) surgical scrub soap to scrub a wound.

- A syringe—35 cubic centimeters (cc) or 60 cc—for wound irrigation. A smaller syringe—6 cc or 12 cc—is useful for eye irrigation.

- Disposable gloves to avoid contaminating a wound with your bare hands. Store these gloves in a baggie to keep them clean before use.

Bandaging Materials

- Topical, water-soluble antibiotic ointment to apply to a wound to keep it protected and moist. Examples include triple antibiotic ointment, silver sulfadiazine cream, and chlorhexidine cream. Avoid using petroleum-based products directly on a wound, especially one that is to be sutured.

■ Sterile, non-stick dressing that is not impregnated with anything, like a Telfa® pad.

■ Roll (Kling) gauze, brown or white—this stretches and conforms to a limb to hold a non-stick dressing or padding in place.

■ Roll or sheet cotton, gamgee, Combine pad, or sanitary napkin to pad the lower leg to prevent pressure on tendons and soft tissues beneath a bandage, or to create a hoof bandage.

■ Self-adhesive stretchable fabric bandage material, like 3-inch or 4-inch Elastikon® or Elastoplast.

■ Sticky elastic, easy-tear bandaging material, like VetWrap® or CoFlex tape, or an ace bandage—these are used for pressure bandaging only when there is sufficient padding on the limb.

■ Bandage scissors with blunt ends.

Other Supplies for Dealing with Wounds

■ Petroleum-based ointment to apply below a wound to limit skin scald from wound drainage, and to lubricate the end of a thermometer.

■ Superglue® to close a small wound until it can be looked at by a veterinarian if there is to be a long delay. Apply it, while holding the wound edges together, as small drops or dabs with sufficient spacing to look like stitches. Keep in mind that this material heats up when applied. Only resort to this if instructed to by your veterinarian due to a potential delay in treatment. Usually, it is best to thoroughly clean and bandage a wound without attempting to close it.

- Flexible rubber tubing or thin strip of leather to use as a tourniquet. Refer to the section on hemorrhage (p. 100).

Additional Items to Consider Including in a First Aid Kit

- A notebook and pen for recording findings (for example, vital signs).

- Rectal thermometer—5-inch mercury or digital for large animals.

- Stethoscope to count heart rate and to check intestinal sounds.

- Needles and syringes if anticipating giving intramuscular (or intravenous) medications. Only administer intravenous medications if comfortable and competent doing so under the advice of a veterinarian, and if okayed by your equine insurance company.

- Multi-purpose tool that includes pliers and a small file. Refer to the section on removing horseshoes (p. 134).

- Tweezers or forceps—for grasping and removing debris, cactus spines, thorns, splinters, or other foreign bodies.

- Sterile saline eye wash solution available at the drugstore for rinsing debris from the eye. Refer to the section on eye injuries (p. 86) for details.

- Fly facemask to keep dirt, bright light, and flies from bothering an injured eye.

- Gorilla or duct tape.

- Hoof pick.

- Hoof boot that has been pre-fitted, usually for front hooves. Trim it so there is no boot contact with the coronary band.

- Fly repellant spray or wipes.

- Flashlight or headlamp with fresh batteries.

- Instant chemical cold or hot packs—cold helps to control inflammation of soft tissue injury. Refer to the section on cryotherapy (p. 126).

- Clean towels.

- Plastic baggies.

Prescription Medications

- Sterile ophthalmic ointment *without* corticosteroid. Do not use eye ointment containing a steroid until a veterinarian confirms that there is no corneal abrasion or ulceration. Refer to the section on eye injuries (p. 86).

- Broad-spectrum oral antibiotics and oral dose syringe. Have a couple days' supply on hand in case there is a delay in access to a veterinarian. Have a veterinarian provide you with instructions on use and follow those instructions. Replenish these supplies when they expire.

- Non-steroidal anti-inflammatory systemic medication (NSAID) in paste, tablet, or powder form—phenylbutazone, flunixin meglumine (Banamine®), or firocoxib (Equioxx®)—to minimize edema, swelling, and pain, and to control fever. Follow a veterinarian's instructions for use. Refer to the section on colic (p. 52) before administering any NSAID to a horse with colic pain.

- ■ Short-acting, sublingual (under the tongue) detomidine sedative (Dormosedan®) for pain relief. This is useful for managing a horse's colic pain or to allow treatment of an uncooperative horse if he sedates well with this medication.

  - • Note: A sedated horse can wake from a stupor and strike out with a sudden and well-placed kick. Stay away from the back end of a sedated horse, and move deliberately, always letting the horse know where you are through voice and touch.

- ■ Dexamethasone tablets or diphenhydramine (Benadryl®) to counteract an allergic reaction. Use only under advisement of a veterinarian.

HOW TO ADMINISTER MEDICATION

How to Use a Paste Oral Medication Without Overdosing or Underdosing

Medications like NSAIDs (non-steroidal anti-inflammatory drugs), Dormosedan gel, and dewormers come with a winder on the applicator that enables you to open the tube sufficiently to provide a correct dose. Usually the tube is labeled with body weight in pounds; other times it is labeled in grams. (Based on the intended, recommended dose, use the horse's body weight or the recommended grams to be given.) Problems develop if the winder is too loose and doesn't hold its place, or if you inadvertently wind it all the way to the end, thereby giving the horse too large a dose or even the entire tube when less is appropriate.

Pay attention when handling medications and know how much you are attempting to give. Don't be distracted while preparing and administering medication. If necessary, place a piece of tape behind the winder located at the exact amount you want to administer. This will prevent the winder from accidentally rolling all the way up and dispensing an incorrect and potentially dangerous amount of drug.

When administering oral medication, make sure the horse's mouth is free of food or debris. Insert the end of the tube along the inside wall of the mouth, then keep the horse's head up and depress the plunger slowly. Work the horse's tongue by massaging it with the syringe—this forces him to swallow the medication instead of holding it in his mouth and potentially spitting it out later.

How to Administer an Intramuscular (IM) Injection

Check the expiration date on every bottle, jar, and syringe before administering medication to a horse. Use a clean needle and syringe for every injection to avoid risk of infection. Never use the same needle on multiple horses—blood contamination can transfer disease as well as infection. Double check the recommended route of administration—should it be given intravenously (IV), intramuscularly (IM), or orally?

When pulling up an injectable medication into a syringe, *read the label three times*—first when you pick up the bottle, again while pulling medication into the syringe, and one last time before you put the bottle down. This helps you avoid inadvertent injection of an inappropriate product. Double check the dose (both amount and concentration) pulled into the syringe.

Return outdated medication, needles, and syringes to a veterinarian for proper disposal. Always wash your hands thoroughly before and after handling medication to avoid skin, eye, or mouth contact from residue on your fingers.

■ The neck is usually the safest place for a handler to access to give an IM injection. Draw a triangle on the neck: The lower "leg" of the triangle runs above the jugular groove and carotid artery; a second "leg" runs in front of the shoulder; and a third "leg" runs beneath the upper neck ligament under the mane.

■ Another common location for an IM injection is along a horse's thigh muscles. Stand well to the side, facing backward, close to the horse's side. It is safer to be in close range; if standing well off to the side, a horse could place a kick with full impact.

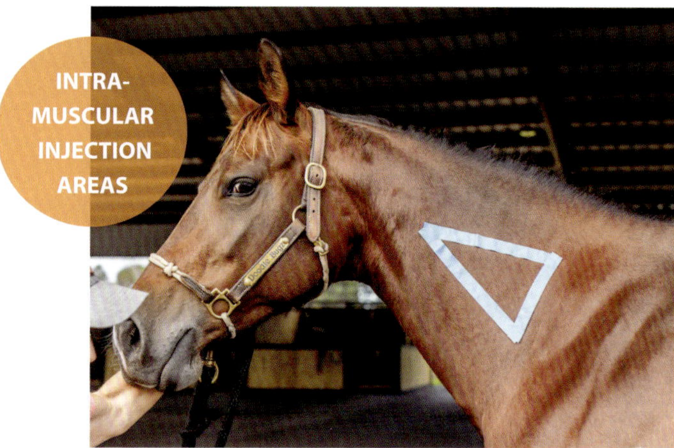

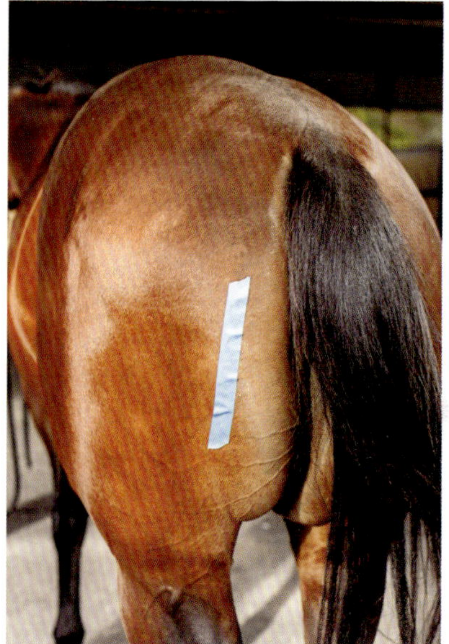

The safe area for an IM injection on the horses neck and along his thigh.

■ Once you isolate the area to use for the injection, place the needle, *without* the syringe attached, into the biggest part of the muscle defined by this neck triangle or along the thigh. Bury it to the needle hub.

■ Once the horse is quiet, attach the syringe, and pull back gently to ensure there is no blood in the needle hub.

■ When you are satisfied that there is no blood, slowly depress the plunger on the syringe to deliver the injectable medication. If you press too quickly, the drug could spurt out the end of the syringe, leaving you administering a smaller dose than intended.

■ If you are administering a large dose, after injecting half the volume in the syringe, pull the needle halfway out and redirect it within the muscle. Check again for no blood by aspirating on the syringe a little, and then proceed to give the rest of the medication.

■ Pull the needle and syringe out in one quick motion. Apply pressure over the injection site for a few minutes if there is blood ooze.

RESPONDING TO AN EQUINE EMERGENCY: GENERAL STEPS

While sometimes difficult to do, keeping a calm mind and demeanor helps when you are faced with an equine emergency. Your horse reads your body language and emotions so if you can keep your composure, that may help him stay calm as well.

Preparation is key to successfully managing an emergency and providing urgent care to your horse in a timely fashion. Prepare by doing the following:

- Know what is normal for each individual horse so you have a mental baseline for comparison when something about a horse seems off to you. If you are aware of how an individual horse usually behaves, and you document information about his normal vital signs, you'll be able to tell when something isn't right. Refer to the section covering assessment of vital signs (see below) for more information.

- Familiarize yourself with common terminology for equine body parts, particularly the legs. This way, you'll be able to communicate clearly with a veterinarian when you need expert help.

- Put your stocked first aid kit with materials and supplies in a place where it will be to hand when you need it. Refer to the section on assembling a first aid kit (p. 17) for details.

ASSESSMENT OF EQUINE VITAL SIGNS

Knowing what is normal for your horse gives you something to compare to his vital signs and behavior during an emergency. Document your findings on paper, cell phone, tablet, or computer. Include the date and time you make each assessment to track progress or deterioration in your horse's condition.

Checking through this list of vital signs won't take very long once you're familiar with the process.

Heart Rate

A horse's heart rate gives you information about his metabolic condition and level of pain. A stethoscope—available inexpensively through on-line websites or a pharmacy—lets you listen to the quality of his heart beats and their rate.

Place the bell end of the stethoscope on the body wall just behind the horse's

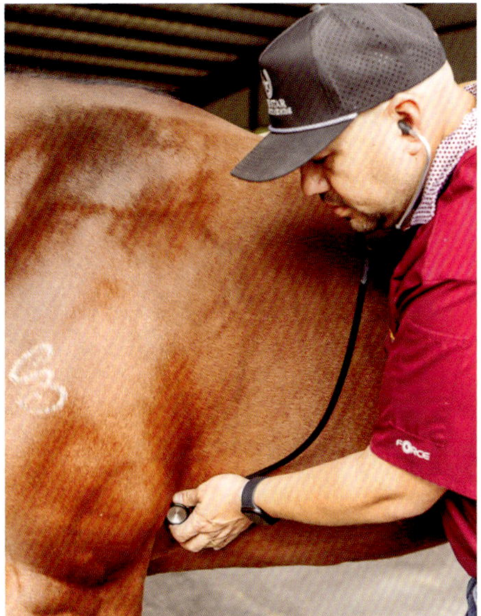
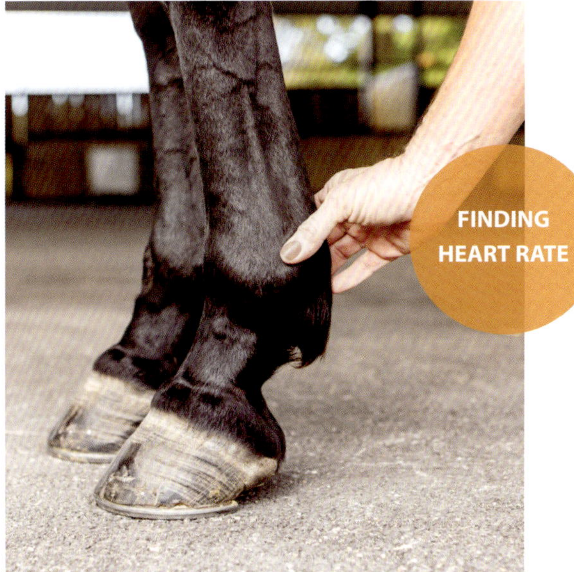

Determining the horse's heart rate using a stethoscope and by feeling the pulse via the rear of a front fetlock.

left elbow, near the bottom of his chest. Listen to each "lub-dub" and count that as one beat. Then count beats for one minute (or count for 15 seconds and multiply by 4). You can also take a horse's pulse by feeling the large artery under the jaw, or the two arteries along the bottom rear part of a front fetlock.

- The normal resting heart rate for a horse is 32–48 beats per minute (bpm). A fit or genetically gifted horse may have a resting heart rate as low as 28 bpm.

- An abnormal resting heart rate is anything exceeding 52 bpm that stays elevated.

  - A horse's heart rate might be elevated during exercise—afterward, though, his heart rate should drop to less than 60–64 bpm within about 10–30 minutes, with the rate of recovery depending on how much and for how long he exerted himself while exercising.

- A resting heart rate up to 64 bpm or higher that persists is a potential sign of pain, anxiety, stress, or illness.

- A heart rate that remains elevated over 80 bpm is usually a sign of a critical condition such as an intestinal twist (torsion) or shock. Pain spasms can cause temporary elevation to this level so you should recheck the heart rate at 10–15-minute intervals to make sure you're getting an accurate picture of the horse's condition.

- A horse with a persistently elevated heart rate often shows other clinical signs of distress at the same time, such as rapid breathing, obvious signs of pain, sweating, and/or distress or depression. (A depressed horse often has a slumped body posture, is not interested in his surroundings, and may also be disinterested in food.) Other parameters are also likely to be affected, such as mucous membrane color, capillary refill time, and intestinal sounds.

Respiratory Rate

Horses normally have a relatively slow respiratory rate. Respirations per minute are evaluated by:

- Each visible diaphragm lift in the flank area is counted as a breath.

- Count each breath exhalation you feel with your hand held in front of a horse's nostrils.

A respiratory rate elevated beyond normal may signal stress or duress, or may be appropriate in high heat climate conditions or when the horse is being exercised.

- Normal respiratory rate in a resting horse ranges between 12–24 breaths per minute.

- Respiratory rate increases with strenuous exercise, fear, or when overheating from fever or heat stress, especially when the temperature and humidity are both high. Refer to the sections on heat stress (p. 71) and fever (p. 64) for details.

- Usually, a horse's respiratory rate is slower than his heart rate. *Panting*—which is medically defined as a state in which a horse's respiratory rate is faster than his heart rate, also known as an *inversion*—is usually associated with heat stress following exercise, or extreme heat and humidity. A panting horse is able to dump up to 15 percent of his heat load through his respiratory tract.

Mucous Membranes

One key vital sign that is an indicator of both metabolic health and the horse's chances for survival Is the condition of the mucous membranes—their color and moistness, as well as how fast they return to their normal color after you press on them (*blanch* them) with a fingertip. You can assess mucous membranes in several places:

- The gums above the teeth, visible beneath a horse's upper lip.

- The underside of the upper eyelid.

- Just inside the lips of a mare's vulva.

Normal versus Abnormal Mucous Membranes

- Mucous membranes should be moist and pink—you can use the pink color you see beneath your fingernails as a visual comparison.

- A pale pink or very pale color is associated with decreased blood circulation, anemia, blood loss, or systemic illness.

- Bright red indicates the horse is in a moderate stage of shock.

- A brown tinge, a gray, blue, or purplish color, or a muddy-looking hue mean the horse is experiencing a life-threatening crisis.

  • Muddy-looking membranes—gray or brown-tinged—indicate very poor circulation, usually due to advanced shock.

  • A purplish color around the edges of the gums along the tooth line, called *margination*, is indicative of *endotoxemia*. The outer cell

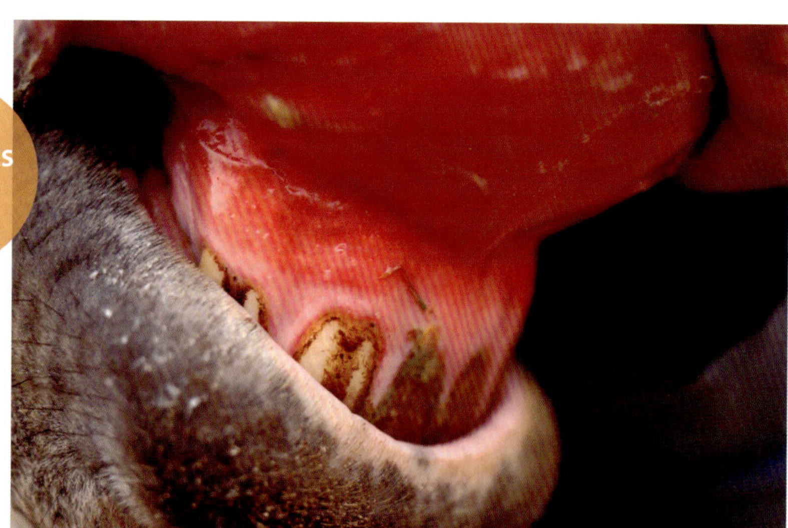

These mucous membranes are brick-red due to cardiovascular shock. This is a very serious and potentially fatal condition.

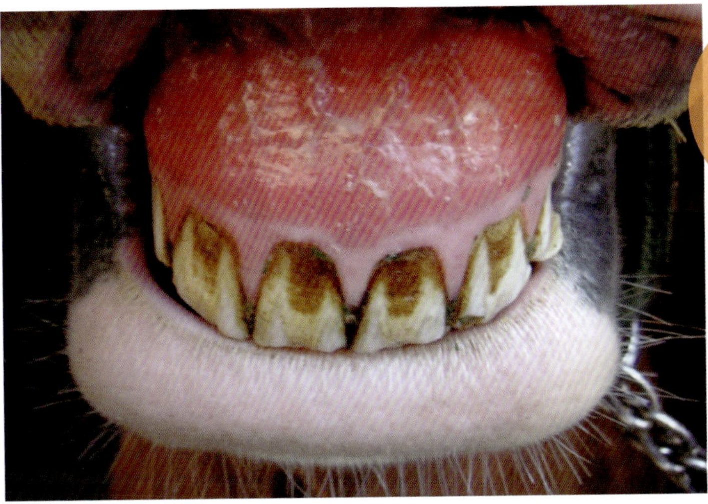

The pale purple just above the gum line is called endotoxic margination due to overgrowth and death of Gram-negative bacteria in the intestines. This creates significant systemic inflammation and needs immediate medical attention.

walls of certain bacteria, specifically *Gram-negative organisms*, are composed of endotoxins. When Gram-negative bacteria die due to intestinal stagnation or bacterial overgrowth, endotoxins are released into the horse's bloodstream, which causes endotoxemia and an associated adverse systemic inflammatory reaction.

A yellow hue (jaundice) occurs with liver stagnation or red blood cell destruction. However, if the horse has recently eaten legumes, his mucous membranes may have a yellowish tinge even though he is perfectly fine.

Capillary Refill Time (CRT)

Capillary Refill Time (CRT) refers to how long it takes the color of mucous membrane to return to pink, following blanching of a horse's upper gum with a fingertip.

- Gums returning to a pink color in less than two seconds is a normal capillary refill time (CRT).

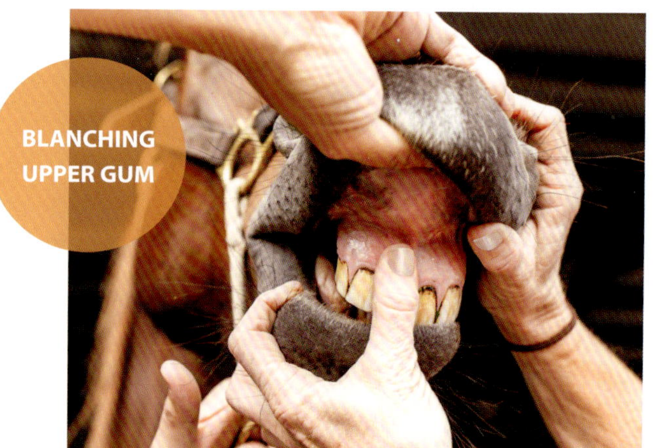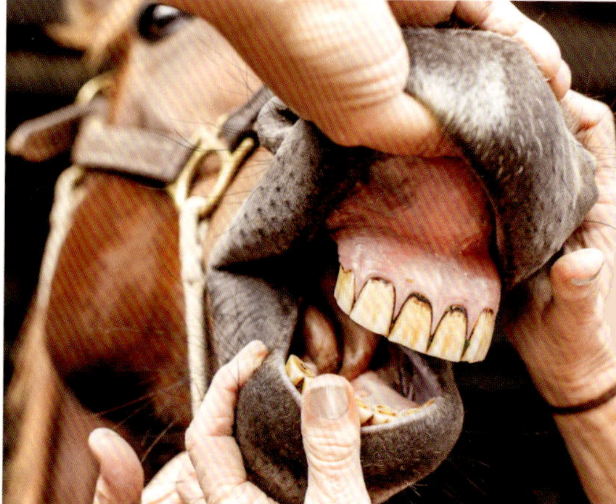

Blanch (press on) the horse's upper gum with a finger, and see how long it takes for them to return to their normal pink color.

- Delayed CRT—more than 2 seconds—indicates a problem with the horse's cardiovascular system, like dehydration, acute blood loss, or sepsis. Refer to the sections on dehydration (p. 40) and shock (p. 69).

Intestinal Sounds

As intestinal contents mix and move through the bowels, you can hear sounds, sometimes with the naked ear and usually with a stethoscope. Listen to both sides of the flanks to assess what is referred to as *progressive motility*, which describes the sounds heard from the normal way ingested food moves through the intestinal tract.

- Listen to the top and lower portion of each flank area on both sides so you cover all four "quadrants" of the horse's bowels with a stethoscope or your ear. The sounds you'll hear when you're listening to the gut of

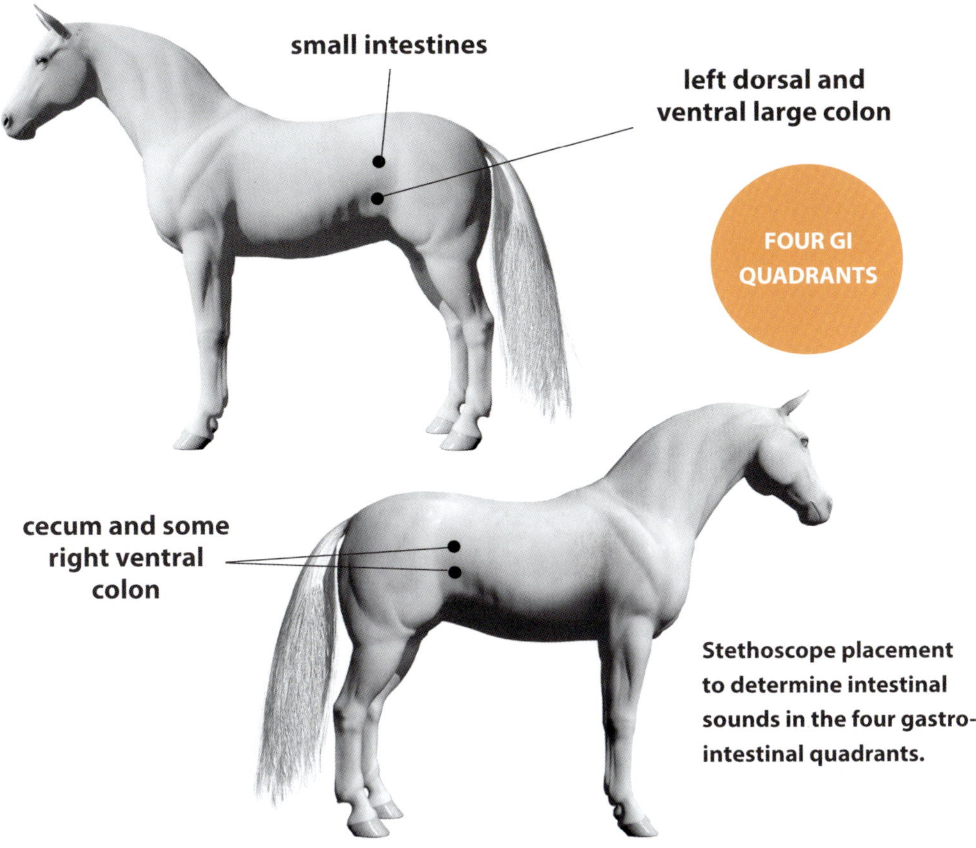

a horse with normal intestinal activity are similar to the rumbles and gurgles of your stomach when you are hungry.

■ It is normal to hear at least two or three intestinal rumbles in each area (quadrant) of the flanks over a couple of minutes.

Abnormal or No Sounds

Decreased bowel activity means diminished intestinal sounds—instead of being digested, food sits in one place and ferments, setting off a domino effect of

Listening for intestinal activity in the upper left quadrant.

problems. It is abnormal to hear no sounds, or only occasional ones, or to hear infrequent sounds that include squeaks or "tinkles" of gas. Some specific sounds indicating specific issues include:

- On the right side of the flanks (over the cecum), sounds similar to a penny falling down a well (tink-tink-tink-tink-tink) are associated with gas in the cecum, likely due to intestinal stagnation.

- Squeaking noises in the bowels indicate that the intestinal tract is trying to move food along (peristaltic contractions are occurring) but normal progressive movement isn't happening.

- Excessive gut sounds could mean that there is an impaction or blockage. Intestinal reflexes increase colon motility in an attempt to move material through the bowel; this results in increased gut sounds.

Loud intestinal sounds may precede complete intestinal shutdown so check the sounds for changes every 10–15 minutes.

■ It is possible to hear the movement of sand in the bowels by placing a stethoscope on the abdominal midline at the level of the girth, near the sternum. You may hear something similar to the sound of roiling surf on a sandy beach, or sand moving in a paper bag. However, the absence of these sounds does not mean there is an absence of sand in the horse's gastrointestinal tract.

■ No intestinal sounds at all—a state called *ileus*—is serious cause for concern. Although there may not necessarily be a physical blockage in the intestines, a quiet bowel is as good as blocked if consumed food or fecal matter is not moving in the correct direction. Absolute quiet and an absence of *intestinal motility* increases the risk of intestinal displacement or torsion, or may indicate that displacement or torsion has already happened.

Bowel Movements

Your horse should have a pretty consistent number of bowel movements each day. Note the number and compare the total from day to day. As a general rule, a horse eating 20 pounds of hay per day often has 18–20 pounds of feces to show for it. Feces contain water, not just solid food waste; so although hay is being processed and nutrients extracted by the intestinal tract, the remaining non-digestible material plus added body fluid just about equals the weight of consumed hay.

Most horses have 8–12 manure movements a day, although this varies depending on the size of the horse and how much he eats. Pay attention to the consistency and quality of the feces. Normal horse "apples" are formed, discrete, moist fecal matter, but not too moist.

- Overly dry manure is firm, with fecal balls that are relatively small in size, small in number, and/or very dark in color. This is most common with dehydration, with a potential for impaction problems.

- A slimy mucous coating is also typical with dehydration and bowel stagnation. The extra mucus that coats dry fecal balls helps to lubricate and move them through the intestinal tract.

- Wet, loose feces can develop if the horse eats too much green grass at pasture, or if his bowels are irritated. Dietary changes, stress, or infection can also upset the intestinal *microbiome* (the bacterial population that normally resides in the intestines), and that can alter manure consistency. Nervous horses or mares in heat may squirt small amounts of loose feces rather than producing a firm pile. These horses should still be monitored since they are losing fluids and electrolytes in wet manure.

- Diarrhea is the production of very wet, often abnormally smelly feces, which may result from a bacterial or viral infection of the gastrointestinal tract, or after serious disruption of the horse's microbiome.

MUCOUS-COATED FECES

This slimy, mucous coating on the feces occurs when there is intestinal stagnation. This is a warning sign that fecal contents are dehydrating and the horse is in need of more fluid to avert an impaction colic.

- *Free fecal water syndrome (FFWS)* is not necessarily abnormal if it doesn't occur along with other problems. FFWS describes a horse that defecates a relatively solid pile of manure, with some wet feces or liquid coming before, during, or after the "normal" manure.

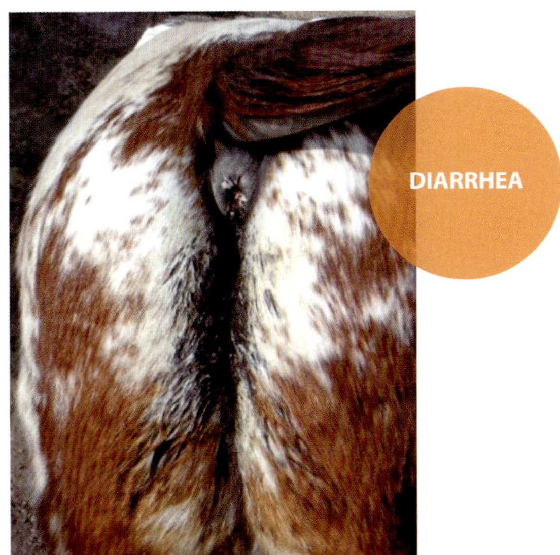

Manure caked under the horse's tail from diarrhea. It helps to clean this up to enable you to monitor for continuing diarrhea or for progress to more formed stools.

Free fecal water staining on rear legs is not always a sign of a problem but should be differentiated from diarrhea.

Urine Output

Check the stall or paddock for areas where a horse has urinated. There should be ample wet spots.

If you have the opportunity, look at the color of the urine as your horse passes a stream. It should be the color of pale straw. Darker yellow means the horse is dehydrated; blood-tinged or red urine is a sign of muscle damage and release of a muscle protein called *myoglobin*. Myoglobin molecules are large; on their passage through the urinary tract, they can damage the kidneys.

In winter, horse urine in snow often appears red due to oxidation of calcium crystals in the urine. Such discoloration tends to be normal and is not necessarily indicative of a urinary tract problem. Monitor the actual urine stream to see if it is pale yellow or tinged red before it hits the ground. If yellow, then all is normal; if red-tinged, it is worth having your veterinarian check things out.

Rectal Temperature

A rectal temperature higher than 101 degrees Fahrenheit in an adult horse or 102 degrees Fahrenheit in a foal is considered a *fever,* which can be a symptom of a variety of problems. If a horse is not behaving normally, or has been traveling, or there has been known or suspected exposure to an infectious disease, it is important to check his rectal temperature at least twice a day.

Rectal thermometers are available as mercury or digital. For adult horses, use a 5-inch thermometer; a human-sized thermometer is appropriate for foals. The thermometer is inserted into the anus for two minutes if it is a mercury thermometer, or until a digital thermometer beeps. It helps to attach it to a string with a clip that hooks onto the horse's tail so you can move safely away from the horse's hind end while you're waiting for the temperature reading.

- A mercury thermometer needs to be shaken down below 96 degrees Fahrenheit before you insert it into a horse's anus.

- Lubricate the thermometer with petroleum ointment or spit.

- Safe insertion of a thermometer is accomplished by facing backward while standing to the side of the horse's hip and lifting the base of his tail. Insert the lubricated thermometer into the anus only if the horse safely tolerates this. It may not be safe to proceed if the horse repeatedly tries to kick. An assistant holding the horse's head should stand on the same side as the person inserting the thermometer so the horse's head can be guided toward both people and the horse's haunches swung away, to avoid a kick. Refer to the section on safe restraint (p. 13).

Normal temperature readings:

- An adult horse has a normal rectal temperature between 97–101 degrees Fahrenheit.

- A foal can have a normal rectal temperature as high as 102 degrees Fahrenheit.

If a horse has other clinical signs such as disinterest in his surroundings (depression) or lack of appetite, any reading above these temperatures in a resting horse is considered a fever.

Horses often have an elevated rectal temperature range of 101–103 degrees Fahrenheit immediately after exercise, especially with protracted or strenuous exertion. Rectal temperature should steadily drop toward a normal range within 20 minutes after the exertion is over, especially if cooling techniques are used, such as application of cool water over large blood vessels and the neck, chest, and legs. Refer to the section on cooling techniques (p. 74) for more details.

- If rectal temperature surpasses 103.5 degrees Fahrenheit, the horse is overheating and needs help cooling down. Refer to the sections on heat stress (p. 71) and cooling techniques (p. pp. 67 and 74).

Hydration

Hydration is important for blood circulation, which keeps tissues and organs supplied with blood and oxygen. You can make a rough estimate of a horse's hydration level by pinching a fold of skin over the point of the shoulder or an upper eyelid, and seeing how quickly it snaps back into position. It should take less than 1–2 seconds to flatten back into place from the pinched position.

If the skin snaps back immediately, this is a normal skin elasticity (*turgor*) response. However, a horse with a normal response may still be dehydrated— the skin won't remain "tented" until a horse has lost 3–5 percent of his body weight. This amount of water loss due to dehydration is a significant enough amount to interfere with performance. Pinching the skin in the right place is important, too—thin, wet, or old horses have less skin elasticity (and less fat) than normal, and even a normally hydrated horse's skin turgor may show a delayed response if you pinch the skin at the neck instead of the point of the shoulder or upper eyelid.

The skin fold pinch test should be used along with other measurements such as heart rate, heart rate recovery, mucous membrane color and capillary refill time, and intestinal activity.

- With mild dehydration (2–3 percent body weight reduction due to fluid loss), a horse often also has a relatively dry mouth and dry mucous membranes.

- Dehydration of 5 percent is associated with sunken-in eye sockets, markedly reduced skin elasticity, and tacky mucous membranes that

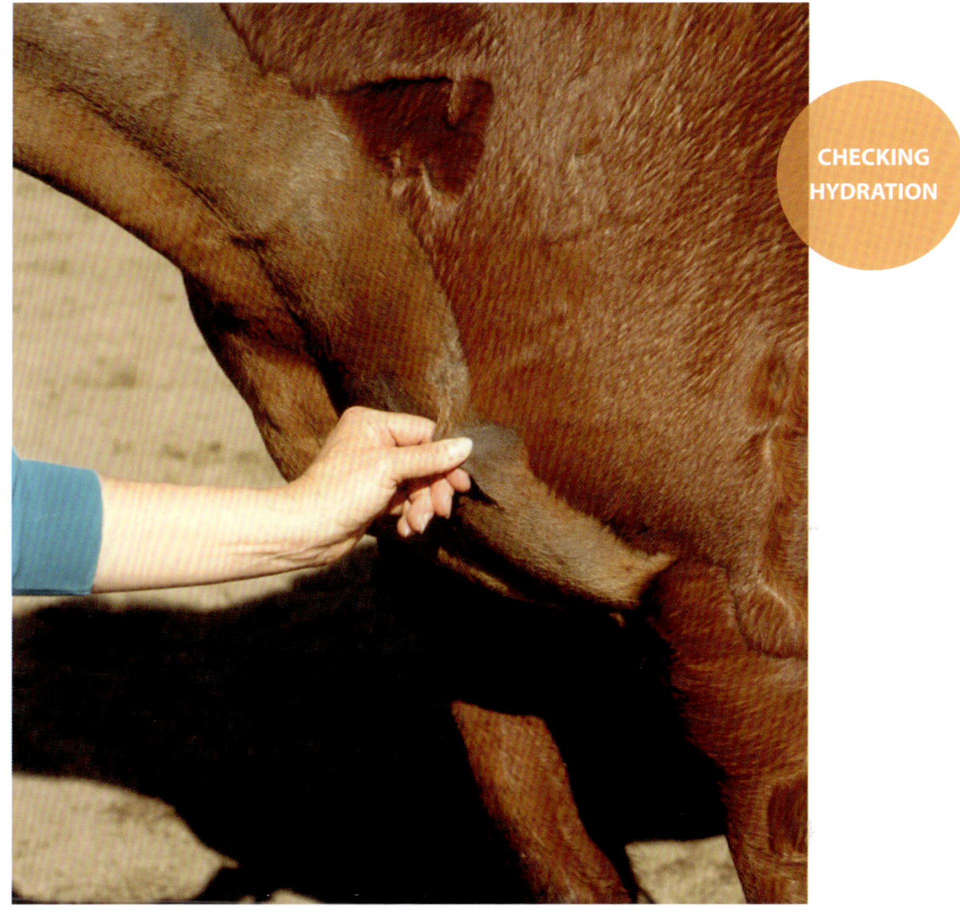

Checking skin elasticity to determine hydration using the "skin pinch" test.

are lacking in moisture. The horse also is likely to display a dull or listless attitude and posture.

- Dehydration of 7–10 percent is serious and life-threatening. Skin turgor is prolonged, and mucous membranes show poor circulation and are often pale, white, or muddy. A horse in this condition will show other significant issues with his vital signs.

Presence and Level of Pain

An additional and important vital sign to assess is *pain*. Pain can result from many causes. When you are examining the horse, try to discern if there is pain, and if so, to what degree is the horse showing it? A horse in pain often displays *facial grimace* visual signs, such as: pursed lips and muzzle tension; low, droopy, or asymmetrically facing ears; withdrawn and intense stare; muscle tightening around the eyes; and dilated nostrils.

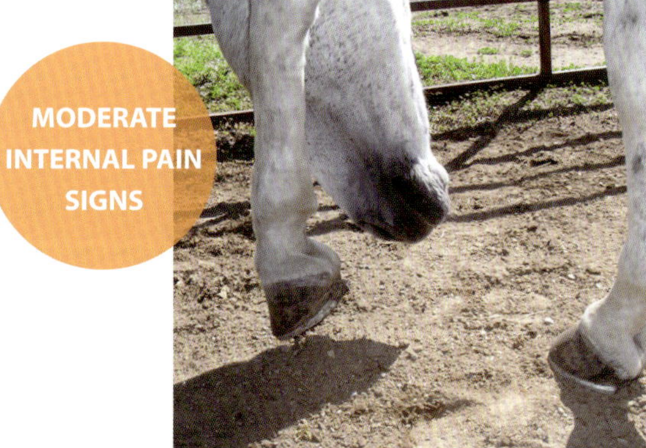

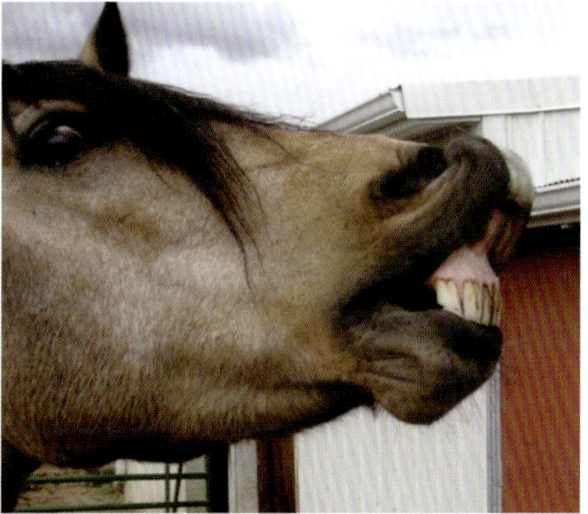

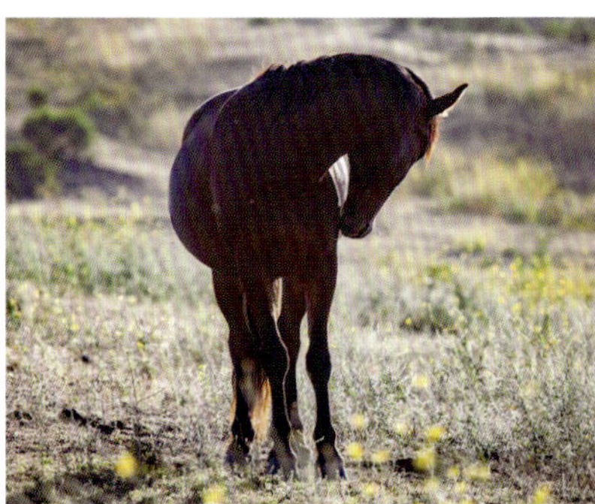

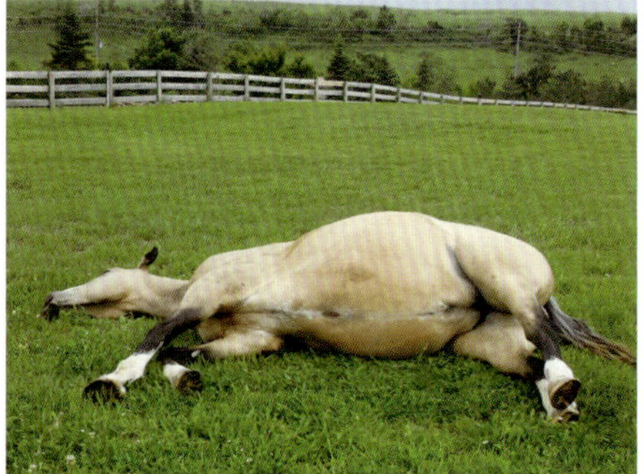

Signs of moderate internal pain: pawing, flehmen response, biting at flanks, and lying down for long periods.

Features of Internal Pain

■ Mild internal pain may cause a horse to be less active, disinterested in his surroundings, depressed, and off his feed, and he might show occasional and intermittent signs of pain such as those described below for moderate pain. Refer to the section on colic (p. 52).

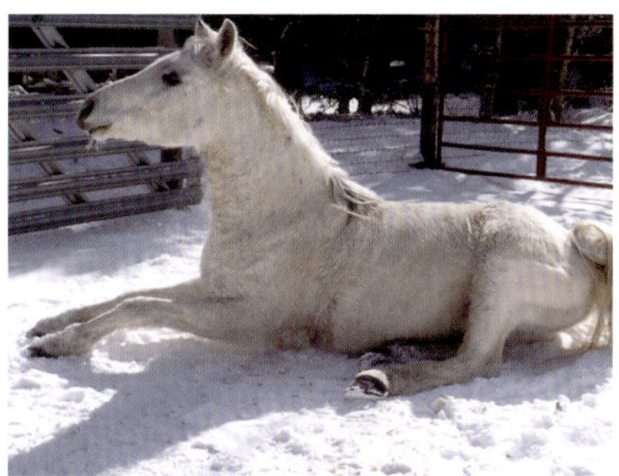

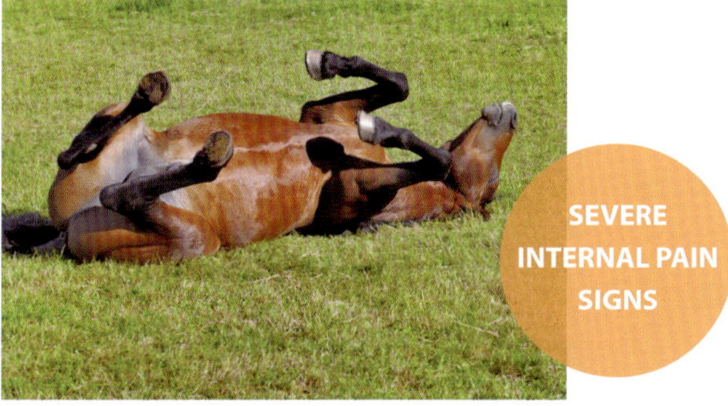

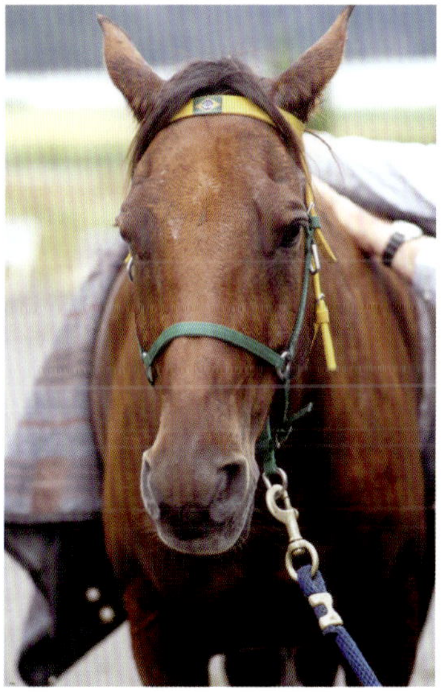

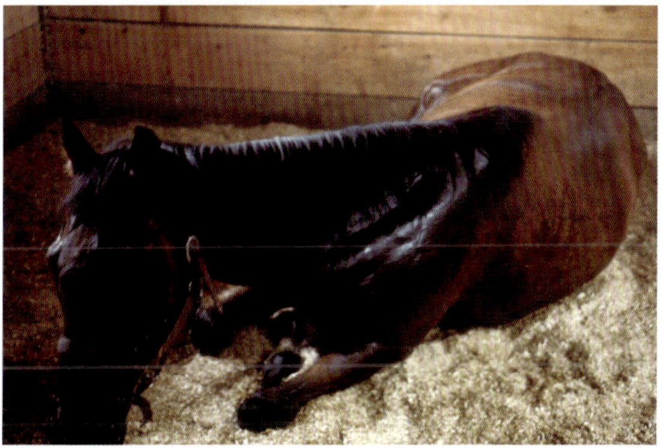

Various signs of severe internal pain: getting up and down, vacant expression with ears back, rolling, and sweating.

- Moderate internal pain causes a horse to be less active, disinterested in his surroundings, depressed, and off his feed, and he may also paw the ground, roll his upper lip (the *flehmen response*), bite at his flanks, kick at his belly, splint his abdomen (tucks up the belly muscles and holds them tight), lie down for unusually long periods, chew wood, or play in his water tank without drinking. Refer to the section on colic (p. 52).

- Severe internal pain may cause a horse to get up and lie down repeatedly because he is unable to find a comfortable position. He may grind his teeth, hold his face in a grimace (with puckered lips and a vacant stare), or he may sweat, thrash, or roll violently on the ground and be impossible to control. Refer to the section on colic (p. 52).

Features of Musculoskeletal Pain

- Mild musculoskeletal pain is often associated with poor performance and lameness, and with the horse shifting his weight from limb to limb, pointing a limb, cocking a leg, or standing in an awkward position. Refer to the section on acute lameness (p. 119).

- Moderate musculoskeletal pain is more obvious as a horse in this state will be reluctant to put his full weight on a painful leg but will still use the limb for ambulation. His gait may be significantly altered because he'll use exaggerated limb movement at walk or trot to relieve pressure on a sore area, or stand in a camped-under position. Some horses bite at the bothersome leg. Refer to the section on acute lameness (p. 119).

- Severe musculoskeletal pain is a possibility when a horse completely avoids putting weight on a limb, acts depressed or colicky, or both. Refer to the section on acute lameness (p. 119).

PART 2

THE SICK OR INJURED HORSE

WHAT TO CONSIDER AND WHAT TO DO

SIGNS SOMETHING MAY BE WRONG

Not all "sick" horses will look the same or do the same things—and each one may be dealing with a different problem. A horse that is acting sick or injured may be off his feed or in pain; he may have intestinal issues or have caught an infectious disease. Let's examine some signs you can look for in a horse that isn't feeling well or may be hurt. *A reminder that what follows are steps to take in the short term while awaiting professional veterinary help.*

POOR APPETITE

How Much Should a Horse Eat and Drink in a Day?

Most adult horses consume about 1½–2½ percent of their body weight each day, which means a 1000-pound horse eats 15–25 pounds of forage per day. Some of this poundage might come in the form of other supplements such as complete feed pellets, grain, fat supplements, or beet pulp. A diet of *at least* 50–60 percent fiber (hay, roughage, pasture) helps the horse's intestinal system function at its best; the higher the percentage of forage, the better.

For every pound of feed he eats, a horse needs 2–4 pints of water for digestion. For example, a 1000-pound horse consuming 20 pounds of food each day needs a minimum of 7.5 gallons (30 liters) of water to process that food. This is the minimum he has to drink just to digest his food; he'll need more water for other bodily functions, and even more for athletic endeavors. The daily amount of water a horse drinks depends on seasonal and climatic conditions, and how hard and long the horse is exercising. Typically, a 1000-pound horse drinks 10–25 gallons of water per day—lesser amounts in winter, considerably more in warm weather, and extra with exercise. Water should never be withheld from a horse.

Horses tend to follow routines in their day. Mealtimes are important to horses that are given specific amounts of food at a certain time of day rather than free choice hay or pasture. When a normally hungry horse is not interested in food, it is definitely time to look for a possible reason. Start by checking your horse's vital signs as described in the section on assessing vital signs (p. 26).

Signs That a Horse Is Not "Hungry as a Horse"

There are times when a horse's appetite is lacking. What are some signs around mealtimes that can tip you off to a possible problem?

- The horse is quieter than normal.

- Instead of a usual greeting at the gate or stall door, he remains withdrawn.

- Rather than interacting with others in the herd like usual, he stands by himself, sometimes in a corner of the field or paddock.

- And, of course, his appetite may be visibly off: a normally avid eater leaves some of his meal behind, picks at his food, eats more slowly than usual, or has no interest in food.

What Causes a Horse to Be "Off" His Feed?

Horses can be very discriminatory about their food. Some may want to eat but only pick at their food; some may have no appetite at all and turn up their noses even when offered the most delectable items. The information you glean from your exam and vital signs check may not reveal an obvious problem. Refer to the section on assessing vital signs (p. 26).

A horse's appetite may diminish due to a variety of problems besides illness or injury, including dental and mouth pain, gastric ulcer disease, and discomfort or pain stemming from the abdomen or musculoskeletal system.

What to look for if a horse is off his feed:

- Signs of pain or discomfort with indications of a possible location or source.

- A rectal temperature reading that indicates a fever. Refer to the section on rectal temperature (p. 38) and the section on fever (p. 64).

If you've been through the entire list of vital signs and still can't identify any other clinical signs besides a poor appetite, investigate further, looking for a systemic illness or problems with the food. Work through a checklist in your sleuthing:

- Problems with the quality of his feed can discourage a horse from eating. Hay or grain that has mold, dust, excessively stemmy material, weeds, or an abnormal odor or appearance often curbs a horse's appetite.

- A horse that eats a little but then starts to cough or gag and is no longer interested in food may be experiencing an episode of *choke*, particularly if green-ish or feed-laden material is spewing from his nostrils. Refer to the section on choke (p. 59).

- Dental issues may cause a horse pain when he is chewing, especially if his hay is stemmy or coarse.

What If a Horse Lacks the Desire to Eat at All?

- Take the horse's rectal temperature to determine whether he has a fever; if he does, he may have caught an illness or be experiencing inflammation and discomfort. Refer to the sections on rectal temperature (p. 38) and also on fever (p. 64).

- Check all of his vital signs, and look for indications of colic pain. A horse may stop eating because of a feeling of intestinal "fullness" due to trapped gas and fluid in a stagnant bowel—this could eventually lead to pain. Refer to the sections on assessing vital signs (p. 26), pain (p. 42), and colic (p. 52).

- How much urine and manure is your horse passing? Refer to the sections on bowel movements (p. 35) and urine output (p. 38), and on colic (p. 52). Scant manure may foretell colic; runny diarrhea may be due to an infection.

- How much water is the horse drinking each day? Refer to the section on how much a horse should eat and drink in a day (p. 46).

- Does the horse have a cough or nasal discharge or have difficulty breathing? Refer to the sections on cough (p. 83), respiratory issues (p. 81), and choke (p. 59).

- If your horse is on any medication(s), consider the possibility that he is having an adverse reaction to a drug. It is also possible that he's experiencing some other non-drug-related allergy.

INTESTINAL ISSUES

If you know what your horse's bowel movements are like when he's feeling well—the frequency, the size and number of fecal balls—you'll be able to tell whether anything has changed when an issue crops up that has you concerned for his health.

Change in Manure Quantity or Consistency

Any change in the amount or consistency of a horse's manure can potentially tell you something about his condition.

- Check his vital signs. Refer to the section on assessing vital signs (p. 26). Pay close attention to his intestinal sounds and mucous membrane color, and monitor him for obvious signs of discomfort— refer to the section on colic (p. 52).

- Monitor his water intake and urinary output. Offer him a bucket of plain water, and another bucket of water supplemented with electrolytes.

- To accurately monitor an individual horse's manure output, stable him in a clean paddock or stall by himself.

- Examine his manure, looking for signs of intestinal stagnation such as feces coated with light-colored gelatinous material (mucus), or signs of dehydration, such as hard fecal balls. If his manure is barely formed, runny, or squirting and watery, or smells unusually bad, this is a sign of diarrhea, discussed in more detail in the following section.

A marked decrease in or absence of manure could signal a potential impaction that can progress to colic signs. Reduced quantity or an absence of manure is a true emergency and it is smart to obtain emergency veterinary care when possible.

DIARRHEA

The horse can also have the opposite problem to having hard, dry, minimal, or absent manure: he passes loose, often liquid feces, referred to as diarrhea. Usually the horse's large colon absorbs up to 30 liters of fluid a day. Any medical condition that interferes with this absorption means a lot of fluid leaving the body instead, creating wetter feces. Diarrhea ranges in consistency from a soft, cow-pie plop to projectile, watery feces. Loose, watery, or extra-smelly feces might mean the horse has an intestinal tract infection or colitis, which can be life-threatening.

What to Do for Diarrhea

If the horse is showing no pain and no abnormalities in his vital signs, diarrhea should improve within 24–48 hours. If it persists longer than that, then veterinary care is necessary.

- Isolate the horse in a dry lot from other horses. Refer to the section on biosecurity (p. 154).

- Clean up diarrhea in the stall and paddock, and from the horse's rump to track the consistency and frequency of his bowel movements.

- Eliminate pasture and all grain products and supplements from the diet, offering the horse only high-quality grass hay.

- Monitor what and how much the horse eats and drinks. Refer to the section on how much a horse should eat and drink in a day (p. 46).

- There are products called oral intestinal protectants that minimize absorption of toxins through the bowel lining—examples include bismuth subsalicylate, activated charcoal, or di-tri-octahedral smectite (Bio-Sponge®). Administer Bio-Sponge® per the manufacturer's directions, or administer 4 ounces of bismuth subsalicylate (Kaopectate® or Pepto Bismol®) every 4 hours by oral dose syringe for up to 2–3 days. Consult your veterinarian for a dose individualized for your horse.

- Administer psyllium added to a small amount of soaked complete feed pellets or soaked beet pulp. Repeat daily for several days to a week, provided the horse continues to improve. Psyllium helps move sand through the bowel if sand irritation is what's causing the diarrhea, and it also serves as a prebiotic to nourish normal gut microbes. Forage also helps move sand through the bowel.

- Provide ample clean, fresh water, and free-choice salt. A horse with diarrhea is losing fluids and electrolytes that need to be replaced. Add 1 ounce (about two tablespoons) of table salt to a gruel of pelleted feed or mashed beet pulp if the horse is drinking well.

COLIC

Colic refers to intestinal pain and cramping. Colic is a clinical sign associated with behavioral changes, not a specific disease. Intestinal pain occurs for many different reasons: Gas or intestinal spasms, impaction, intestinal displacement, or a twisted loop of bowel referred to as a *torsion*.

Signs of Colic Pain

Clinical signs of colic vary from mild to severe, and variations in between.
The horse:

- Is lethargic, depressed, or disinterested in his surroundings or other stimuli.

- Has an absent or decreased appetite.

- Plays in the water tank but is not really drinking.

- Looks at one or both flanks while acting uncomfortable.

- Displays a *flehmen response* (curling of the upper lip) in response to discomfort or pain.

- Paws the ground as a sign of distress.

- Kicks at his belly, stretches out, or both.

- Lies down and stays there, or gets up and lies down repeatedly.

- Rolls on the ground, especially repeatedly, and not because he is having a body scratch.

- Appears anxious or distressed; paces or walks around intermittently or continuously.

- Shows facial expressions of pain, like grimacing, holding his ears back, or having a vacant stare.

Additional signs of colic:

- Sweating.

- Muscle fasciculations (trembling).

- Distended abdomen.

- Trauma to the horse's head, body, or both, including damage around the eyes and face, due to violent rolling.

- The horse is covered in mud or shavings from rolling, and there may be damage to walls or fencing.

Non-Intestinal Causes of Colic Signs

Non-intestinal issues may cause a horse to display colic signs when, in fact, his intestines are just fine:

- Tying up (myositis or muscle cramping).

- Pleuropneumonia.

- Choke.

- Painful laminitis.

- Dental pain.

- Beginning stages of labor in a foaling mare.

What to Do for Colic

Keep a calm mindset, and work to figure out how serious your horse's bellyache may be. Note that a horse in the early stages of a serious colic may not yet have a high heart rate or dramatic pain. Initially, he may only show disinterest in his surroundings and loss of appetite, play with his water without drinking it, or curl up his upper lip (flehmen).

Every case of colic is unique and each horse's ordeal must be addressed individually. Your friends' past experiences have little relevance to what your horse may currently be experiencing. Waiting for hours to see if colic pain resolves is counterproductive—and dangerous for the horse's well-being and odds of survival.

- Check your horse's vital signs and assess any behavioral clues. Refer to the section on assessing vital signs (p. 26).

- Encourage a prone horse up to a standing position and see if he'll stand quietly.

- Once off the ground, the horse may appear okay for a bit and then become uncomfortable again. As long as he has no musculoskeletal issues that preclude exercise, put him on a longe line, or set him free in a round pen or an enclosed arena. Ask for a vigorous trot for about 10 minutes. The trotting motion may move and release gas bubbles, which will resolve a simple gas or spasmodic colic.

- Following this exercise, if there is no improvement in his condition, consider a trailer ride to see if that helps; if not, then you can continue on to veterinary care or call for immediate help.

What to Do for a Recumbent Horse with Intestinal Pain

■ Always keep yourself out of harm's way by positioning yourself behind the recumbent horse, away from the swing arc of his legs and head.

- Encourage a recumbent horse to rise off the ground. This may require a definite effort. A horse that refuses to get up is often in significant pain, possibly but not necessarily due to "colic," as in the non-intestinal examples listed on p. 54.

Then, check all the horse's vital signs to try to figure out what is going on. Refer to the section on assessing vital signs (p. 26). If the horse is behaving erratically or violently, do not put yourself in harm's way.

What About Rolling?

There's a persistent and pervasive myth that if a colicky horse isn't allowed to roll, then he won't develop an intestinal twist. Actually, this is not the case—a horse can be standing upright and still develop an intestinal *torsion* (twisting of the intestine on its axis) that requires surgical intervention.

If the intestines lack normal motility or are distended with gas or accumulated intestinal contents as with an impaction, then this abnormal motility may pull the bowel out of position, causing a displacement. A displacement may be just that—a section of bowel that has migrated to an inappropriate place in the abdomen—or it may be a full-blown torsion, which means the intestine has rotated on its axis, or an *intussusception,* where the intestine telescopes inside itself.

Rolling may increase the chance of displacing a loop of bowel, particularly when intestinal motility is compromised, but many colicky horses roll without suffering such a serious problem. In some cases, they are even able to self-correct a mild displacement with rolling.

What Else to Try

If you try the trot technique described on p. 55 but the horse is still uncomfortable or disinterested in eating, allow him to rest quietly if he lies down again. It is counterproductive to walk a horse with colic pain hour after hour, as was done in many decades past. It is best for both the horse and handler to conserve energy by allowing a horse to rest quietly if he will.

However, a horse that is thrashing and rolling violently can inflict harm to himself, his handler, and other bystanders. In that case, get him up and walk for short periods as a distraction. Keep yourself in a space where you can escape being trapped or injured. It is advisable to get veterinary care to a very painful horse as quickly as possible.

Resist the Temptation to Medicate with NSAIDs

Medicating a horse with colic with a paste form of *non-steroidal anti-inflammatory drugs (NSAIDS)*—for example, *flunixin meglumine (Banamine®)* or *phenylbutazone ("bute")*—can create a whole host of other problems, and these pastes should be used cautiously, if at all, for multiple reasons:

- Oral medication is poorly absorbed by the intestines of a horse with poor gut motility, which is often the case with colic. Even under normal circumstances, oral medications require several hours to be absorbed fully—an oral dose is less likely to help with immediate colic pain, and once given, interferes with both a veterinarian's assessment and the ability to administer medication intravenously to provide immediate pain relief.

- ■ NSAIDs are powerful and may significantly mask the symptoms of a problem that actually requires surgery, thereby delaying appropriate treatment.

- ■ NSAIDs can cause kidney function problems and even gastric or colonic ulcers in a dehydrated horse.

- ■ Injectable flunixin meglumine, given intramuscularly, can cause an anaerobic *Clostridial sp.* muscle infection, with life-threatening consequences.

In addition, the label dose of flunixin meglumine is *twice* the amount that should be given to a colicky horse—such a large dose is able to mask a serious condition for as much as half a day. This could delay appropriate medical and surgical intervention, and reduce the horse's chances for survival.

Other Medication Options for Pain Control

There are other medications that are appropriate for helping with colic pain.

- ■ A short-acting sedative provides pain relief and muscle relaxation, including in the smooth muscle of the intestines. An oral product, *Dormosedan gel (detomidine)*, is available with a veterinary prescription. It is applied along the underside of the horse's tongue. This drug is *not* meant to be swallowed. Rapid absorption through the mucous membranes allows sedation to take effect within 15–20 minutes. However, a horse may not obtain relief if his unrelenting pain is due to a potentially surgical condition.

- ■ *Dipyrone* provides mild pain-relieving effects. Because of that, this medication doesn't tend to mask escalating pain.

■ Another medication that does not mask escalating pain is *Buscopan*®, which, thanks to its antispasmodic action and relaxation of smooth muscle, can help alleviate spasmodic colic pain. (The horse's heart rate may accelerate for 30 minutes following administration of Buscopan®.)

However, either dipyrone or Buscopan® must be given intravenously (IV) and *only* administered by those comfortable and competent with IV injections. If your horse is insured, check with the insurance provider before administering any intravenous medications—should something go wrong, above and beyond the intestinal danger to your horse, this may nullify your coverage.

CHOKE

When we think of *choke*, we think of food material trapped in the back of the throat or in the airways, the same way it is trapped when humans choke. However, in horses, the food material is trapped in the *esophagus* because it is either too large an amount, or too dry to be swallowed. Horses that bolt their feed and those fed pelleted feed are the ones most prone to developing choke. Dehydration also reduces the saliva available to help the horse swallow his food successfully.

Here's what you might see in a horse affected by choke as he attempts to relieve the blockage:

■ Green, frothy, mucus- and food-laden material oozing or spewing from the horse's nostrils.

■ Repeated gagging and coughing.

■ Repeated stretching of the head and neck.

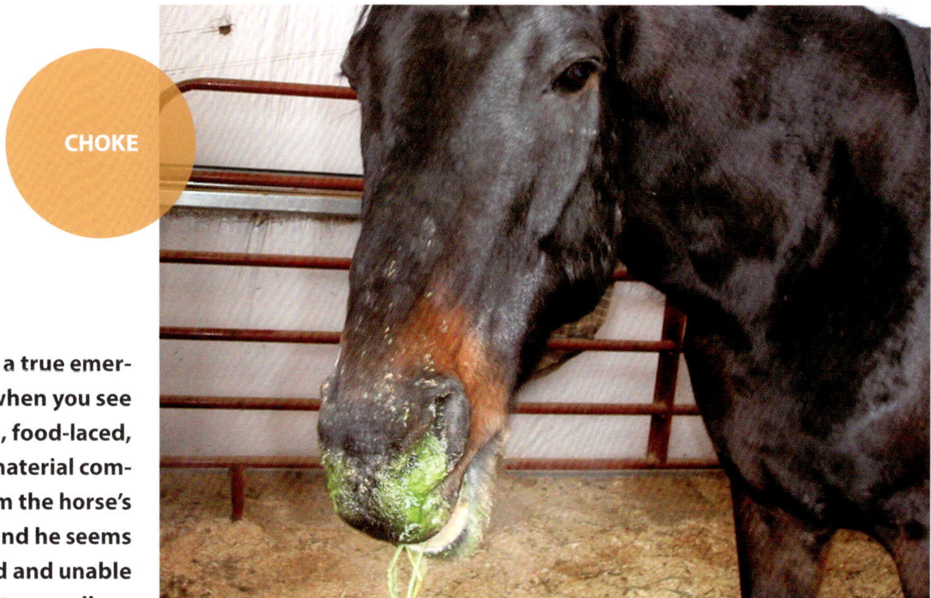

Choke is a true emergency when you see green, food-laced, frothy material coming from the horse's nose, and he seems distressed and unable to eat or swallow.

■ Distressed or colicky behavior, even to the point where the horse will throw himself on the ground. Some choking individuals are very dramatic.

One danger of choke is development of *aspiration pneumonia*, from inhalation of feed material and saliva into the lungs as the horse coughs and gags.

What Can You Do to Help?

■ If there is a slight slope available, position the horse with his head down to help lessen the risk of inhalation of food, saliva, and mucus.

■ If available, with veterinary advisement, administer:

• A short-acting sedative (*Dormosedan gel*) that relaxes the horse and drops and lowers his head—this helps lessen the risk of aspiration.

Whole-body relaxation as well as relaxation of esophageal smooth muscle might allow the choke to spontaneously resolve.

- *Oxytocin* is useful to relieve esophageal spasms associated with obstruction.

- Any sedative (*xylazine* or *detomidine*) or oxytocin given by intravenous injection should be administered only by those comfortable and competent with IV injections.

Don't give the horse food or water until it is clear that an episode of choke is entirely resolved. Veterinary intervention is often necessary to relieve choke in a horse by passing a stomach tube and irrigating and softening the obstruction with water. In some cases, intravenous fluid therapy is necessary to hydrate the mass obstructing the esophagus.

Follow your vet's guidelines on how to manage the horse once the choke has been resolved. A wet mash or gruel eases the passage of food down an inflamed esophagus for days. For prevention, pre-soak pelleted feed with water to form a gruel or mash prior to feeding, or place large rocks in the horse's feed bucket to slow him down when he eats.

GRAIN OVERLOAD

Not all horses need to be fed grain, especially those in only light work and low-level athletic pursuits, but many owners like to have some on hand to offer as a treat. It is best to have a feed area specifically designated for grain and rich foodstuffs (alfalfa or other legume hay) that can be locked up securely so it isn't accessible to a horse that gets loose on the premises.

It isn't always obvious that a horse has gotten loose, as he may return to his paddock once he's eaten his fill. The presence of piles of manure scattered around in areas where they shouldn't be is a tell-tale sign that one or more horses accessed areas of the property that are normally off limits.

A carbohydrate (grain) overload is a life-threatening condition and requires immediate veterinary attention.

- Over-fermentation of grain starch in the intestines causes overgrowth and death of bacteria, with release of *endotoxin*—the substance that makes up the cell walls of *Gram-negative bacteria*—into the blood. Systemic changes and abnormalities in blood circulation in the limbs that occur with grain overload can lead to crippling *laminitis* in the hooves. Refer to the section on laminitis (p. 136).

- Excess gas in the bowel from starch fermentation can cause colic. Refer to the section on colic (p. 52).

- The highly fermentable nature of grain (or mowed grass clippings) can cause the stomach to rupture.

How Much Is Too Much Grain?

- Ingestion of even 4–5 pounds of grain can be an issue for some horses.

- Consumption of 15–25 pounds of grain in one short period is dangerous.

It is often hard to tell exactly how much a horse has eaten. Even if scattered grain doesn't look like much, it is best to assume the worst. Assume that even a less dominant horse overindulged once dominant horses ate their fill and moved away. Treat all horses that could have had access to the grain, even if you think one horse is low in the pecking order and didn't get an opportunity to eat too much. The risk to an untreated horse that does need help is life-threatening.

Timing and Strategies of Treatment

- If the condition is treated aggressively within the first 8 to 12 hours, most problems associated with grain overload can be averted.

- Optimal treatment involves veterinary intervention such as stomach tubing the horse with mineral oil or activated charcoal, which limits endotoxin absorption and reduces gas fermentation. Additionally, the veterinarian will administer anti-inflammatory medications and apply frog support to the hooves to protect against laminitis.

- If you can't get immediate professional veterinary help, then under direct advisement from a veterinarian, administer a non-steroidal anti-inflammatory medication (NSAID) like flunixin meglumine (Banamine®) or phenylbutazone.

- Another potentially helpful strategy is to ice the hooves prior to the development of overt laminitis pain. You'll need to immerse the horse in ice water or ice sleeves up to the knees. Ideally, icing should be applied as much and as consistently as possible for the first 24 hours. If ice is unavailable, immersing a horse's legs in a cold stream is useful.

FEVER

A horse may be off his feed or lethargic because he has a fever.

What Causes an Elevated Rectal Temperature?

Fever develops for many reasons, including infectious disease, sepsis, and heat stress.

- Check vaccine records to ensure your horse is up-to-date on infectious disease immunizations, especially those for respiratory infections, mosquito-borne viruses, tetanus, and rabies.

- Think about which kinds of insects your horse might have come into contact with, keeping in mind your geographical location and the time of year.

  - Ticks carry *Lyme disease*, which is caused by *Borrelia burgdorferi* bacteria. A horse with Lyme disease may have multiple symptoms that won't necessarily make it easy to narrow down a diagnosis: Low-grade fever, shifting limb lameness, muscle tenderness, muscle wasting and weight loss, stiff gait, lethargy, behavioral changes, increased sensitivity of skin to touch, and uveitis (inflammation of the eye tissues surrounding the pupil). Joint swelling can occur but it's less common in horses than in dogs and people. Rarely, an infected horse may experience neurologic signs, referred to as *neuroborreliosis*.

  - Ticks also carry *Anaplasma phagocytophilum* (previously referred to as *equine granulocytic ehrlichiosis*), which infects white blood cells.

Symptoms include a high fever (over 104 degrees Fahrenheit), low appetite, depression, *limb edema* (swelling), *petechial hemorrhages* (tiny blood spots on mucous membranes like the gums and inner tissue of the nose), *icterus* (*jaundice*—a yellow hue of mucous membranes), and reluctance to move due to muscle soreness or a lack of coordination (*ataxia*).

- *Eastern or Western equine encephalitis* viruses are carried by mosquitoes. These viruses cause a variety of neurologic symptoms. An infected horse develops a fever, involuntary muscle twitching, and an ataxic (uncoordinated) gait. Increasingly severe symptoms of encephalitis develop, such as head pressing, aimless wandering, seizures, hyperexcitability, and coma. Eventually the horse goes down, unable to rise. Refer to the section on neurological syndromes (p. 146). While Eastern equine encephalitis is increasing in incidence in recent years, Western equine encephalitis is not currently a problem but could become active once again with climate change.

Horses infected with *West Nile virus (WNV)* develop a variety of neurologic signs that occur in different combinations: depression; stupor; fever; ataxia; limb weakness and stumbling; partial paralysis; inability to stand; muscle twitches; muzzle tremors; and facial paralysis and other assorted signs related to the cranial nerves. Horses with severe neurologic effects may not regain the ability to stand, and may experience convulsions or blindness. Refer to the section on neurological syndromes (p. 146).

- Consider recent travel and competition history as that might inform you of the potential for an infectious disease outbreak, such as equine herpesvirus, strangles, or viral respiratory disease. Consult the Equine

Disease Communication Center (EDCC) for alerts on recent outbreaks (equinediseasecc.org/alerts).

- Have new horses entered the property without going through a quarantine period? Even if a horse shows no sign of sickness, he can be a carrier and bring disease onto the property. Refer to the section on biosecurity (p. 154).

- Does the horse have a swollen leg or legs? Is there an associated wound? Refer to the sections on wound care (p. 97) and lameness (p. 119). If you see "stocking up" (*limb edema*) in multiple legs, the horse may have contracted a systemic disease like *Equine Viral Arteritis (EVA)* or a secondary reaction to the strangles bacteria that is developing into *purpura hemorrhagica*. Or, leg swelling may be due to circulatory stagnation in limbs that were unprepared for the exercise demands of the day. It is important to differentiate exercise-related stocking up from a systemic disease.

- Is there nasal discharge or cough? Refer to the section on respiratory issues (p. 81).

- Is there diarrhea? Refer to the section on diarrhea (p. 51).

In general, a horse with a fever appears lackluster and won't have much of an appetite. He may have rapid breathing and an elevated heart rate. Check his rectal temperature, and refer to the section on the topic (p. 38).

A rectal temperature higher than 101 degrees Fahrenheit in an adult horse or higher than 102 degrees Fahrenheit in a foal corresponds to a fever, especially when there are other signs of potential problems showing up at the same time.

An exercising horse typically develops rectal temperatures of 101–103 degrees Fahrenheit, but this steadily subsides to normal range usually within 20–30 minutes once exercise has stopped. A horse experiencing heat stress also breathes rapidly and has an elevated heart rate. See the section on heat stress (p. 71).

Consequences of Fever

A fever is a warning sign that the horse is experiencing some kind of infection or heat stress. A fever is not usually harmful unless it is prolonged, high, or accompanied by other signs of a problem. In addition, a febrile horse often stops taking care of himself, foregoing food and water. This means he has the potential to develop dehydration and then impaction colic.

- If a horse's fever elevates above 103.5 degrees Fahrenheit, he needs help cooling down. Refer to the section on cooling techniques (see below).

- A fever over 106 degrees Fahrenheit can be life-threatening, and can even cause convulsions or seizures, although this is rare.

- Isolate a horse with fever or illness from other horses to curtail an infectious disease outbreak as much as possible. Follow biosecurity strategies to limit exposing other horses on the property. Refer to the section on biosecurity recommendations (p. 154).

Cooling Techniques for Fever

What can you do to help cool your horse down when he is experiencing a high fever or heat stress?

Techniques to cool a horse rely on the same principle as relieving internal heat with sweat: evaporative cooling.

- Move the horse to an area out of direct sunlight. Choose areas of shade with fresh, moving air.

- Using a water-soaked sponge or towel, soak the horse's neck and chest repeatedly with room-temperature or cool water. Scrape off excess to remove warmed water, and reapply. Continue this procedure until the horse's chest feels cool to the touch, or rectal temperature drops below 103.5 degrees Fahrenheit. Then stop and monitor rectal temperature every 10–15 minutes. Take care not to cool down a horse too quickly.

- Soak only the large muscle areas and the neck and legs *in front* of the withers. Except under special circumstances, avoid applying water to a horse's entire body because rapid cooling of the large haunch muscles can lead to muscle spasms or chilling. See the section on tying up (p. 77).

- However, in very hot and humid climates, a whole-body soak may be necessary to help lower a horse's internal temperature. Scrape water away, and continue to apply more until the chest feels cool to touch or rectal temperature falls below 103.5 degrees Fahrenheit.

- If the horse's fever persists, it may be appropriate to administer non-steroidal anti-inflammatory (NSAID) medications. Consult with a veterinarian before medicating. Use caution when medicating a dehydrated horse with NSAIDs, as this medication can increase the risk of kidney damage and gastric ulcers.

DEHYDRATION OR SHOCK

Mild dehydration of as little as 2–3 percent is associated with a decrease in performance. A horse can dehydrate this much just by traveling a long distance in a horse trailer, especially when the weather is hot and humid. Protracted exercise also leads to mild or moderate dehydration.

If exercise continues and a horse develops more significant dehydration, serious metabolic problems can occur, associated with obvious clinical signs. Significant dehydration and cardiovascular compromise can cause a horse to develop shock. Refer to the section on hydration (p. 40).

What to Look for in a Dehydrated Horse

Check all vital signs to determine if a horse is in metabolic trouble that could lead to shock. Refer to the section on assessing vital signs (p. 26) for all these parameters. Dehydration and shock are associated with many of the following clinical signs:

- The horse's heart rate remains elevated above 60–80 bpm.

- His respiratory rate may be rapid and panting—or it may not.

- His mucous membranes are tacky and abnormal in color: pale, muddy, purplish, or brick red.

- Capillary refill time is delayed beyond 2–3 seconds.

- His skin, when pinched at the point of the shoulder or the eyelid, remains tented for a prolonged time, beyond 1–2 seconds.

- The horse is depressed and not responsive to his surroundings or stimuli.

- The horse is off his feed.

- With shock specifically, the horse's ears and muzzle may be cool to the touch due to poor blood circulation to the extremities.

Note that moistness of the gums and a skin pinch test are only basic assessments of hydration status and can't always tell you whether a horse is dehydrating further.

How to Get a Horse to Drink

We are all familiar with the adage, "You can lead a horse to water, but you can't make him drink." Losing too much sodium chloride (electrolytes that combine to form salt) in his sweat during protracted exercise interferes with a horse's normal thirst reflex, even when he actually needs to drink the most. Here are some tricks that might stimulate a horse to drink:

- Offer him water in several different types of buckets—galvanized, rubber, and plastic. A choice of different materials may encourage drinking from whichever bucket is made of the horse's preferred material.

- Offer him a bucket of plain water, and a separate bucket of water that contains dissolved electrolytes.

- Offer him a wet, sloppy gruel of pelleted feed or beet pulp soaked in water. Add ½–1 ounce of table salt only if there is ample water in this mixture.

- Soak his hay with lots of water.

- Allow the horse to graze on green grass, which has a high water content. Don't allow grazing for too long if he's unaccustomed to eating green pasture.

- While this isn't the right place to start in the face of a crisis, it's a good idea to train a horse in advance to drink water laced with cider vinegar or Gatorade®, which disguises anything odd about the taste of water from an outside source.

HEAT STRESS

Heat stress generally develops due to overexertion leading to overheating rather than to external heating by the sun's rays. A horse that takes a long time to recover to normal heart rate after exercise, is panting with flared nostrils, has a rectal temperature greater than 103.5 degrees Fahrenheit, or has any combination of these signs is likely suffering from heat stress.

Signs of Heat Stress

If you spot any of the following signs, it is time to rest the horse and use the cooling techniques described on p. 74:

Movement

- Flagging body posture under saddle.

- Unwilling to maintain forward momentum or speed without rider urgings.

- Flattened stride.

- Poor impulsion.

- Ataxic (incoordination) or weak movement, including stumbling.

Attitude and Posture

- Grumpy disposition when handled.

- Grumpy when asked to perform.

- Lack of alertness or interest in surroundings.

- Dull or glazed eyes.

- Sagging or deflated posture at rest.

- Wrinkled lips.

- Ears at half-mast.

- Anxious expression.

Body Functions

- Waning or absent appetite.

- Lack of thirst.

- Reduced or absent urination.

- Reduced or absent bowel movements.

- Decreased intestinal sounds.

Overt Problems

- *Tying up syndrome* (*myositis*, muscle cramps).

- *Thumps* (*synchronous diaphragmatic flutter*)—the diaphragm contracts with each heartbeat, a state associated with electrolyte imbalances.

- Colic.

- Neurologic signs—lack of coordination (ataxia), poor awareness of surroundings or stimuli.

A horse can develop dehydration and heat stress during hot and humid weather conditions, especially when ridden in difficult terrain, or for protracted periods or at speed in any conditions, or when hauled in a horse trailer for long periods during very hot weather. Under any of these circumstances, it is important to continually monitor a horse's vital signs. Refer to the section on assessing vital signs (p. 26).

In addition to the vital signs above to evaluate for an exercising horse, another important indicator of how well a horse is coping with exercise is heart rate recovery:

- A horse undergoing aerobic exercise for prolonged periods, such as in endurance sports, should have his heart rate drop to less than 64 bpm within 10–20 minutes once exercise stops. His heart rate should continue to decline to a normal range within 30 minutes, and at most, within an hour.

- You can also use the *Cardiac Recovery Index (CRI)* to assess an exercising horse: Take a baseline heart rate. Trot the horse out 125 feet and back 125 feet—this trot distance usually takes around 30 seconds. At the start of the trot, start your stopwatch. At exactly one minute, take the heart rate again. It should be the same or lower than the starting heart rate. For example, if the starting pulse is 64, then we like to see the one-minute pulse at 64 or 56 or lower. If it's higher, as for example 64/68 or 64/72, that may point to underlying metabolic issues, including dehydration.

Cooling Techniques Following Exercise

Cooling techniques can be found in the section on fever (p. 67). However, for the exercising horse, a few added strategies will help you cool the large muscle groups to relieve the body heat that develops with movement. Repeatedly (every 10–15 minutes) monitor the horse's progress by measuring vital signs and heart rate recovery.

- Slow the horse to a walk for several minutes.

- Dismount and remove all tack, equipment, or blankets, but leave a halter on. If the weather is windy, cold, or wet, a horse could rapidly chill. In that case, cover the rump with a light sheet, blanket, or clothing garment.

- Continue walking the horse; this allows blood flow to continue to flush metabolic waste products and heat from the horse's muscles. Bringing a horse to a sudden and complete standstill after moderate to strenuous exercise causes blood to pool in the muscles, which decreases the amount of blood circulating through his body, and contributes to relative dehydration without helping him cool down.

- Shade is important to both comfort and cooling. Find a shaded area with good air circulation, preferably with a light breeze. Fans are helpful for convective cooling—which means air flows across the horse's body to pull heat from his skin.

■ Periodic, short walks help the horse's muscles pump heat away from deeper tissues.

■ Copiously bathe the horse's head, neck, armpits, and legs with cool water. Large blood vessels in these locations carry heat to the surface of the horse's skin, and repeated soaking helps with evaporative cooling. Sponge and soak him while walking him and when he is at rest until he is adequately cooled.

■ Continuously apply and scrape water away until the horse's skin feels cool to the touch. Don't drape wet towels over his head and neck and leave them in place; towels insulate, so they'll only trap his body heat against his skin instead of allowing it to escape.

■ Heat normally radiates from the head to keep the brain cooler than the inner core temperature of the body; any increase in heat to the brain contributes to central or mental fatigue. Bathe the horse's head as well as the large blood vessels in his neck (jugular veins and carotid arteries) and legs to help move heat out of the central body core.

■ Cooling down an overheated horse too rapidly can cause chilling or muscle cramps (tying up, myositis). Decrease body temperature by about 1–2 degrees Fahrenheit over 30–40 minutes.

• In hot and humid climates, ice water may be applied to the horse's entire body with less risk of muscle cramping.

• However, ice water baths in drier climates can cause problems in large muscle groups—blood vessels will constrict farther away from the surface of the horse's skin while retaining metabolic by-products and heat that need to be carried out of the muscles' depths. In that case, not only will the horse have more trouble recovering from exertion, but also he might develop tying up syndrome, with painful muscle spasms. In arid climates, it is best to limit cooling baths to areas in front of the withers. Refer to the section on tying up (p. 77).

■ Monitor rectal temperature and muscle tone as you cool off the horse. Once his rectal temperature reaches 101–102 degrees Fahrenheit or his chest feels cool to the touch, you can pause or stop cooling techniques. Continue to monitor his rectal temperature for another 10–20 minutes.

■ Offer the horse water to drink. For horses exercised at gallops or sprints, start out only offering small, frequent drinks. In contrast, allow horses working at aerobic paces to drink as much as they want.

Heat Exhaustion

■ If a horse is severely overheated—to the point of clinical heat exhaustion—he may need rapid cooling by any available means, including full body immersion in a pond or creek, or pouring buckets of water over him or hosing and soaking his whole body.

■ A horse in a serious heat stress crisis also needs immediate veterinary intervention with intravenous fluids to avoid shock.

MYOSITIS OR TYING UP

Tying up syndrome, or *myositis*, describes a muscle cramp that typically occurs in the haunch or thigh muscles but can occur in any large muscle group, including the back, shoulders, or neck. Such cramps are often related to dehydration, electrolyte depletion, heat stress, or a combination. In unusual cases, muscle cramping is associated with influenza virus or hormonal changes such as estrus in a mare, or may be due to a metabolic disturbance or muscle disorder like equine *polysaccharide storage myopathy (PSSM)*.

Signs of Myositis

- The horse shortens his stride.

- There is a noticeable change in his disposition or willingness to work, with the horse requiring constant encouragement to keep working.

- The horse is suddenly lame in one or both back legs, with lameness ranging from subtle to severe.

- The horse refuses to move.

- The horse's muscles feel firm or the horse reacts with pain to firm hand pressure over the muscles of the haunches or along the thighs.

- Colic-like signs develop, including sweating, overt pain, rolling, and a rapid heart rate.

- The horse's urine may be discolored or dark. This is because of *myoglobin*, which is a large protein released with muscle damage,

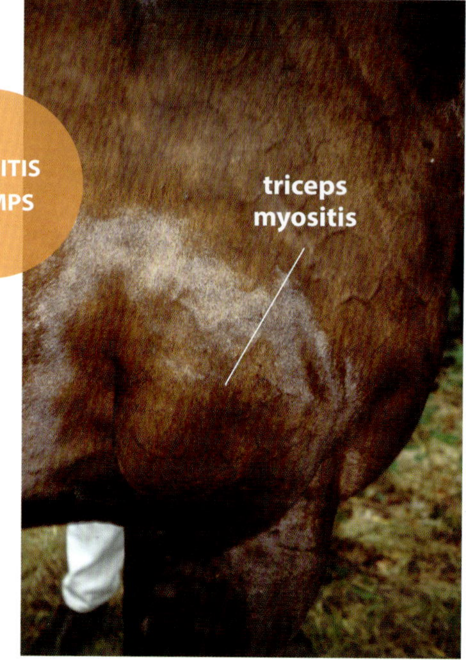

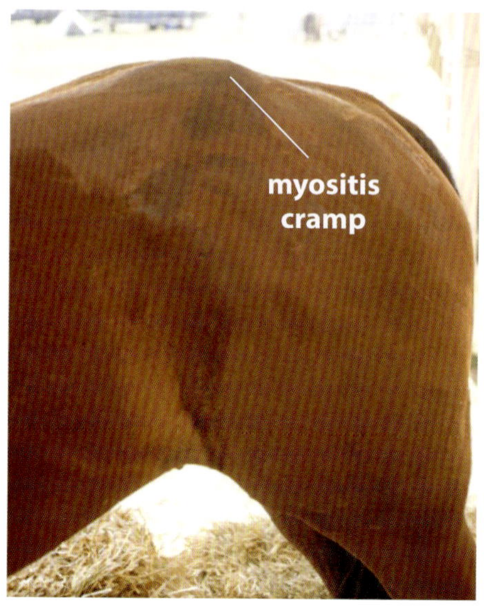

Here you can see a myositis cramp in a shoulder muscle (left) and gluteal muscle (right).

referred to as *myoglobinuria*. However, stiff and cramping muscles are not always accompanied by myoglobinuria.

No matter the reason or the severity, you should immediately stop working a horse that you think might have myositis. Other steps to take to limit further muscle damage:

- Dismount and move the horse to a safe area with sufficient space for him to lie down if he decides to.

- Pull off the saddle, bridle, and gear, but leave the halter and lead rope.

- If there is a cool chill or breeze, or wet weather, cover the cramping muscle(s) with a saddle blanket or light jacket.

This red-tinged urine stream is caused by the breakdown of muscle proteins (myoglobin) when a horse experiences myositis (tying-up or cramps) due to dehydration and electrolyte imbalances. Myoglobin is a large muscle protein molecule that has the potential to cause kidney damage as it tries to pass through the kidneys.

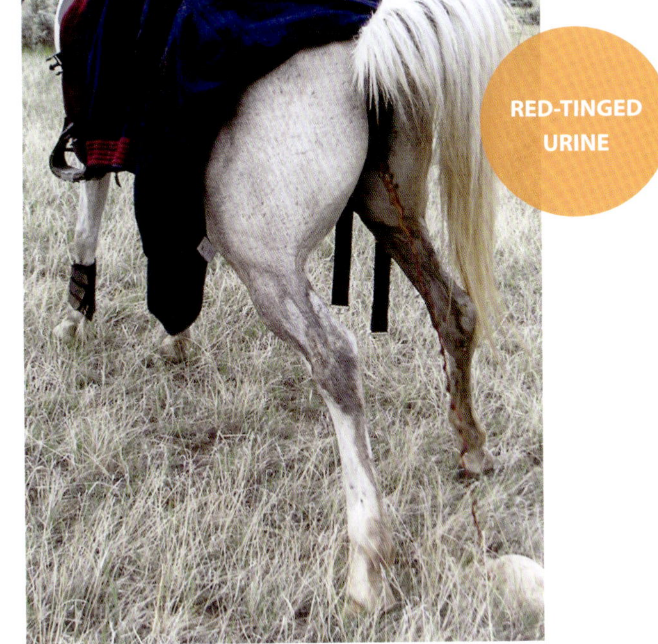

- Allow the horse to graze, rest, and drink water.

- Provide oral electrolytes when the horse drinks if he has been exercising for prolonged periods.

- Refrain from deep muscle massage to avoid adding to muscle damage.

- If the horse is overheated, apply the cooling techniques described in the section on heat stress (p. 74). Keep water off cramping muscles in the hindquarters, restricting water soaks to areas in front of the withers unless neck or shoulder muscles are also cramping.

- Take it slow with frequent stops to rest as you make your way to the barn. If the horse is not willing to move, arrange for a horse trailer to pick him up to move him to an appropriate location for treatment.

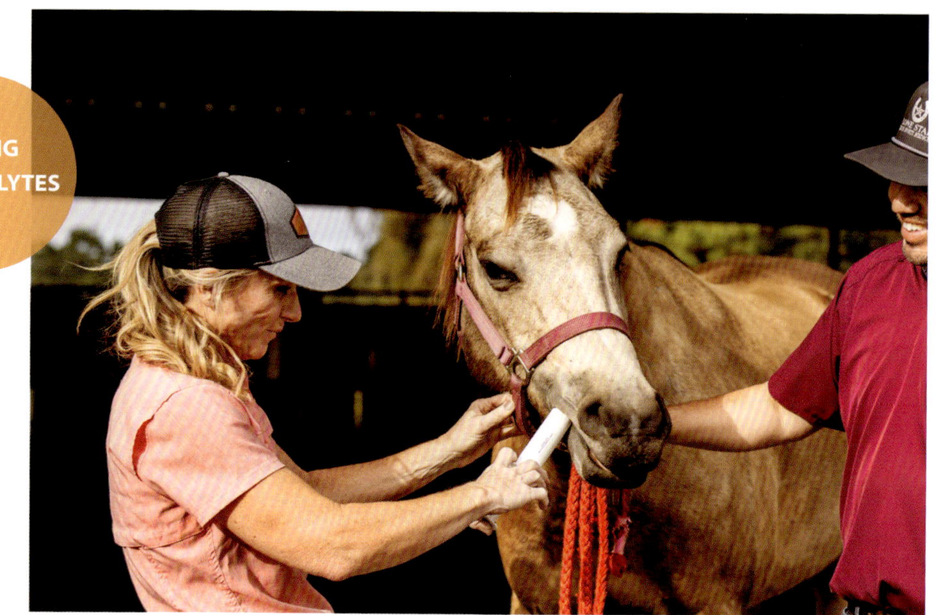

Giving electrolytes via a dosing syringe.

Things to Watch For

- Monitor the frequency and appearance of urination—dark or discolored urine is typical of myositis, and means the horse should receive intravenous fluids to protect his kidneys from damage from myoglobin and dehydration.

- Monitor his gait—stiffness or lameness often coincide with a bout of myositis.

- A horse with myositis may display signs similar to colic. Check his vital signs to help you identify clinical signs that differentiate myositis from colic. Refer to the sections on assessing vital signs (p. 26) and colic (p. 52).

■ Only administer NSAIDs such as phenylbutazone or flunixin meglumine (Banamine®) with caution, and only under veterinary advisement, as these can cause kidney damage or gastric ulcers in a dehydrated horse.

In many cases of myositis, a horse needs oral and possibly intravenous fluids to combat dehydration and flush myoglobin and toxins from the kidneys. This requires professional veterinary care.

RESPIRATORY CONCERNS

A horse can develop respiratory issues that aren't urgent but are related to infectious disease like equine herpesvirus or strangles, which require rapid intervention and biosecurity procedures to prevent an outbreak on a farm or at an event. A horse with respiratory disease or fever should be isolated from others immediately, and kept isolated until he is evaluated and tested and a determination is made that it is safe for him to mingle with others on the farm. Refer to the section on biosecurity recommendations (p. 154).

Nasal Discharge

■ A clear, watery nasal discharge may be normal during exercise or when the horse is eating hay, especially if the hay is dry and dusty.

■ An opaque, white nasal discharge of mucus is a sign of airway inflammation or allergy. This type of discharge may not be particularly serious, unless the horse also shows other clinical signs of a problem like cough, fever, or swollen lymph nodes under the jaw or throatlatch, which could indicate a viral or bacterial infection.

■ A yellowish (pus) or green-tinged (feed) nasal discharge is likely related to an infection or crisis:

- A viral respiratory infection like *rhinitis*, which develops from a secondary bacterial infection.

- Bacterial infection of the upper or lower airways. A common bacterial infection occurs from *Streptococcus equi sp.*, referred to as *strangles*.

- A sinus infection in the head.

- A tooth infection that is draining through the sinus and out the nose.

NASAL DISCHARGE

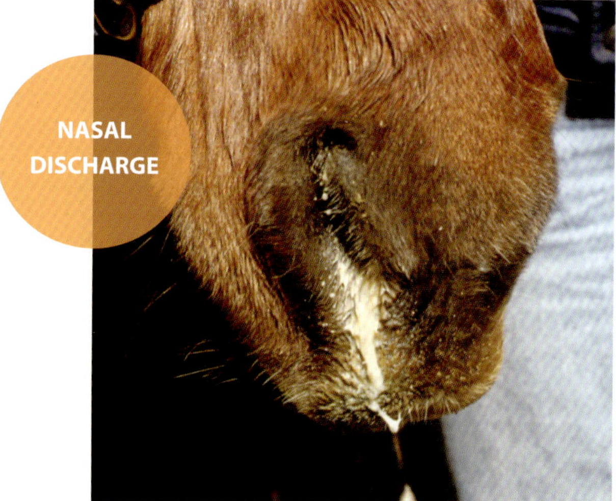

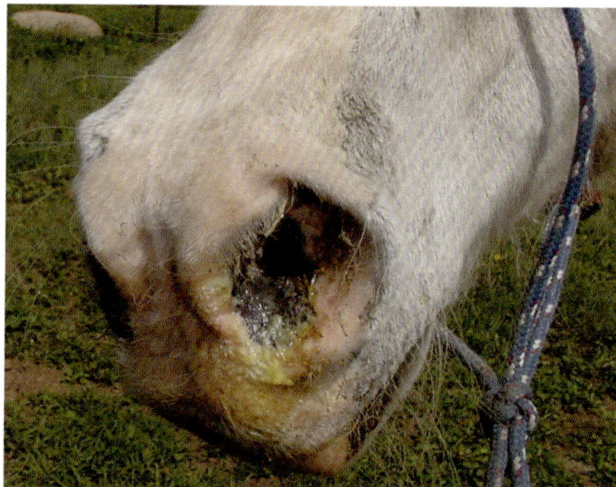

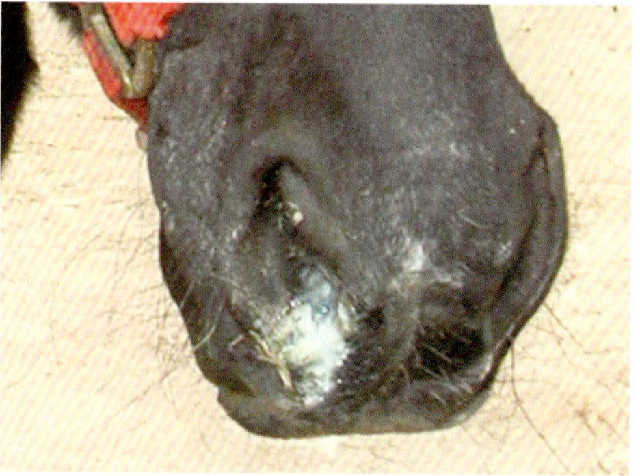

Nasal discharge that is purulent and creamy usually indicates a bacterial infection.

- Choke, if the discharge is laced with food and green material, and the horse is gagging and expelling saliva, food, and mucus from the nostrils. Refer to the section on choke (p. 59). A small amount of green-tinged discharge may be food contamination from the back of the throat that is mixing with normal discharge as a horse coughs. This is different from choke.

Coughing

A horse coughs as a normal reflex to clear debris or mucus from his airways. A viral or bacterial infection can also cause a cough, as does choke. Another possible cause of a cough is *equine asthma*, which is often related to allergies—to dust, mold, endotoxin, and pollen, for example—affecting the lungs.

How can you figure out what is causing a horse to cough?

- Check all of his vital signs. Refer to the section on assessing vital signs (p. 26).

- Check for discharge from the nostrils or eyes, and observe its appearance. Refer to the previous section on nasal discharge (p. 81).

- Does the cough sound dry, or is it wet or expelling discharge or other material?

- Is the horse coughing only when he eats, or only when he exerts himself? Or does he also cough while he is at rest?

  - Have you recently gotten a new batch of hay? Or, are you feeding him old hay from the back of the stack, or from an area that was wet from rain or moist ground and may be moldy?

- Equine asthma often worsens with exercise, when eating dry hay, when a horse is exposed to a dusty environment, or a combination of these.

- Horses with more severe cases of asthma tend to cough for no obvious reason even when at rest.

■ Is the horse able to eat and swallow food? If not, then:

- He may be sick and off his feed. Check his rectal temperature, and refer to the section on assessing vital signs (p. 26).

- He may be experiencing choke; refer to the section on p. 59. With choke, the horse will probably cough and gag persistently, have copious amounts of green material frothing from his nose, and act distressed.

■ Does the horse have a normal appetite and disposition? If not, check his rectal temperature and for any signs of pain or distress. Refer to the section on assessing vital signs (p. 26).

■ Does the horse have a fever or have trouble breathing? These may be signs of an infection, such as *pleuropneumonia* or a viral respiratory disease.

What to Do to Alleviate a Horse's Respiratory Irritation

Once you have checked the horse's vital signs and eliminated choke or an infection as likely causes, you can use a few different management strategies to help ease irritation that is causing a horse to cough.

■ Check hay and forage for mold, dust, or debris.

■ Shake out all the hay to remove as much dust as possible.

■ Prior to feeding, soak the hay thoroughly with water to decrease dust and irritants. You can also steam hay in a commercial hay steamer prior to feeding to lower allergen levels. When a horse is eating dry hay, dust levels can be up to 30–40 times higher in the breathing zone—the air around his nose—than it is in the rest of his stall; soaking or steaming both help with this. You can also feed him low-dust food products, including pellets, quality hay cubes, or haylage.

■ Feed the horse from the ground rather than in hay nets or chest-high feeders.

■ If your veterinarian advises it, treat the horse with a bronchodilator.

■ Refrain from storing hay overhead or in adjacent stalls; moving hay around near stabled horses for feeding stirs dust and particulates into the air.

■ If the horse's cough is mild and not associated with infectious disease, and he can be ridden, ride him outside or in an area with minimal dust kicked up by him or other surrounding horses. You can water the arena before you ride to decrease the amount of dust.

■ Stable the horse outside to provide good ventilation. Particulate levels in an indoor stable environment are usually very high, especially during feeding and stall cleaning. Environmental contamination from those activities can last a couple of hours—and it can be as high as 12–15 milligrams/cubic meter, measured within the horse's breathing zone, which is much higher than the limits the Occupational Safety and Health Administration (OSHA) sets for safe dust exposure levels for humans.

If you suspect the horse has an infection due to cough, nasal discharge, swollen lymph nodes, or fever, then his respiratory crisis could be contagious. Take measures to prevent an outbreak:

- Isolate a coughing horse as far from other horses as possible. Follow practical biosecurity recommendations (see p. 154).

- Seek professional veterinary assistance to examine the horse and perform appropriate diagnostic testing to determine the cause of the cough or other respiratory issues.

If a respiratory problem is due to an infection or severe asthma, once treatment has started, give the horse a minimum of three weeks of rest and recovery before riding him to allow inflammation to subside and give his lung tissue time to heal.

EYE INJURIES

Painful Eye

There are a number of telltale signs of eye pain or injury that will alert you to a problem that needs immediate attention:

- The horse is squinting or holding the eye closed, and seems especially sensitive in bright sunlight.

- The eyelashes are pointing downward—this often happens to an affected, painful eye.

- There is a weeping discharge of clear or opaque appearance from one or both eyes.

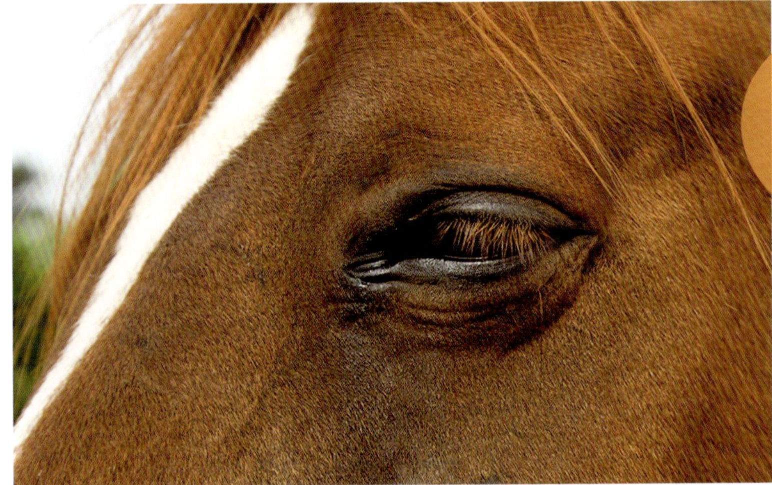

EYE SQUINTING

Eye swelling and squinting occurs from pain and also sensitivity to light (photophobia).

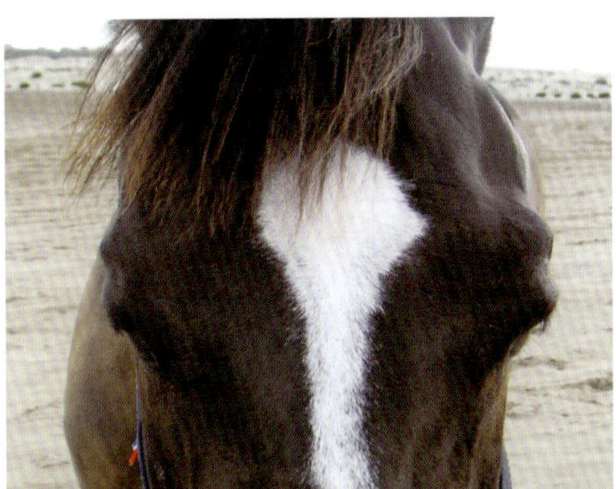

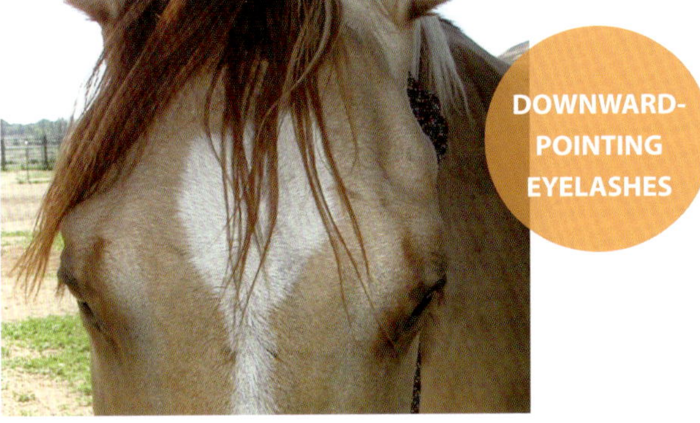

DOWNWARD-POINTING EYELASHES

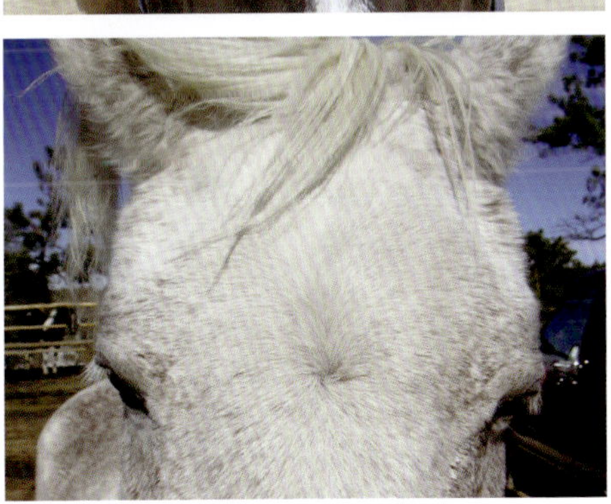

Eyelashes point downward in a painful eye. Compare the clear difference between the gray horse's unaffected eye (on the reader's left) and his painful eye (on the reader's right).

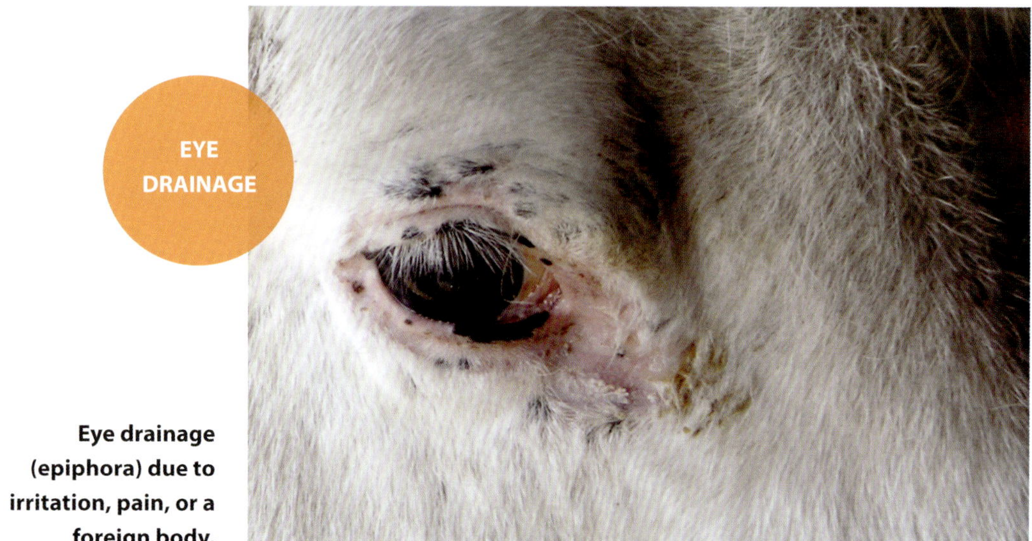

Eye drainage (epiphora) due to irritation, pain, or a foreign body.

- There is swelling and redness in the tissues around and within the eye, such as conjunctivitis.

- The eye looks cloudy or bluish.

Corneal Ulcer

A corneal abrasion or scratch is a common eye injury in horses. Horses run into things, and also dust and debris can collect in their eyes. A break in the tough *corneal epithelium*—an *ulcer*—can be quite painful.

Even a seemingly mild eye injury can turn into a serious problem. Bacteria or fungi that invade the eye can cause an eroding ulcer of the cornea that could turn into vision loss or even loss of the eye. Rapid medical care makes all the difference in shortening healing time and returning the eye to function as quickly as possible, along with easing pain and improving a horse's comfort.

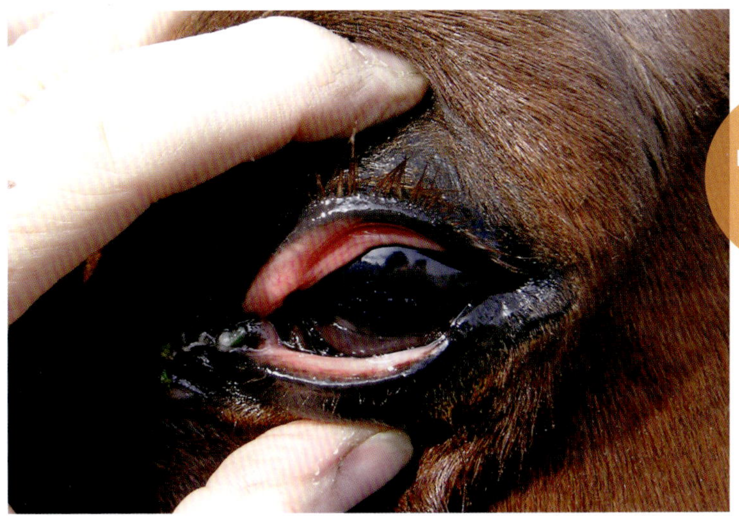

REDNESS IN TISSUE

Redness in the tissues around the eye can indicate conjunctivitis.

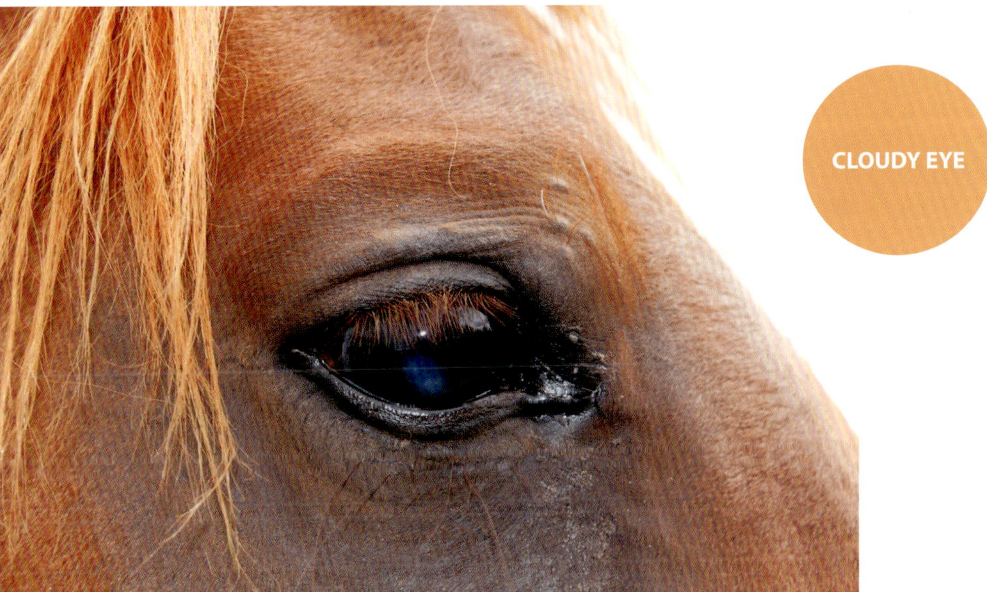

CLOUDY EYE

Cloudy appearance to an eye is often due to corneal edema from a corneal ulcer. It can also be due to an abscess or foreign body in the eye.

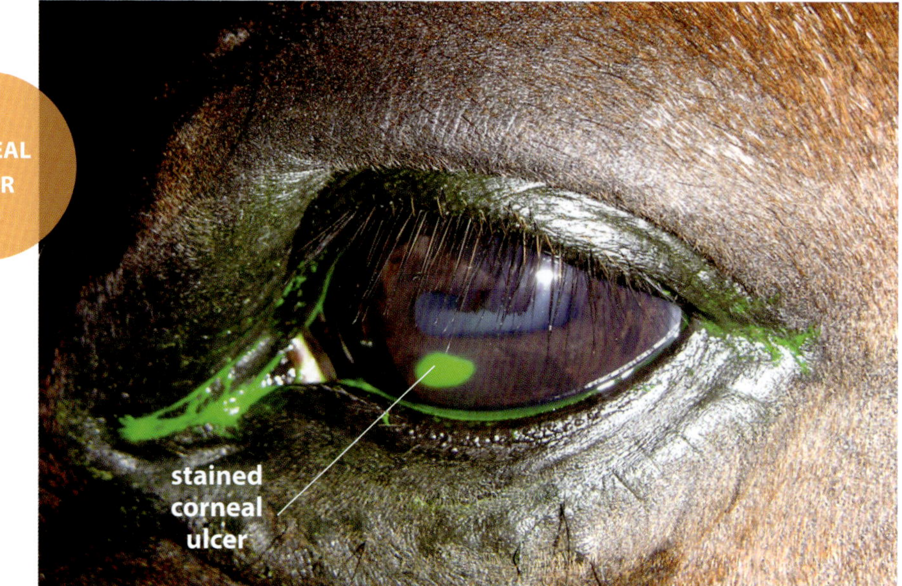

A corneal ulcer is outlined well with fluorescein stain uptake (bright green).

What to Do for an Irritated or Injured Eye

- Rinse out the eye with saline solution to loosen debris or a foreign body. Sterile saline is available on the supermarket shelf in the section with contact lens supplies. You can also prepare a saltwater solution (saline) with ½ tablespoon of table salt dissolved in a quart of clean water. Gently irrigate the eye with a syringe to produce a gentle stream of saline fluid to loosen a piece of adhered hay or flush out debris. Refer to the section on wound care (p. 97).

- Apply antibiotic *ophthalmic ointment* (or drops) specifically intended for use in the eye. Do **not** use any eye ointment that contains a corticosteroid (usually the names of these kinds of ointments end in "–one") prior to evaluation by your veterinarian, as this will worsen a corneal ulcer.

- Broad-spectrum antibacterial eye ointments or drops **without corticosteroids** may be applied every 2–3 hours to medicate and to give relief.

- Ophthalmic lubricating ointments intended for human use (such as LacriLube® or Muro 128), available over the counter, may substitute for antibiotic ophthalmic ointment to give the horse some relief until more appropriate antimicrobial or antifungal medications are available to you from your veterinarian.

- General-use wound medications that are not designated specifically for use in the eye should **never** be used in the eye, as they can cause serious chemical burns. Do **not** use any product intended for external wounds in a horse's eye.

- Use a fly face mask to limit ultraviolet glare, keep flies away, and provide comfort. Check beneath the mask twice a day to make sure no other problems have developed, especially if the horse is rubbing the eye.

- Fly repellants—roll-ons or sprays—should be kept far away from the horse's eyes to avoid chemical burns.

- Monitor the horse to make sure he isn't rubbing his eye excessively against solid objects even with a mask in place.

How to Medicate an Eye

- Hold the medication tube in your fingers, and rest the flat of the palm of that same hand lightly against the horse's face. This allows your hand to smoothly follow any movement of the horse's head instead of leaving you stabbing blindly with the medication tube—and potentially poking the horse (or yourself) in the eye.

- Use the thumb and index finger of your free hand to gently pry open the horse's eyelids.

- Gently squeeze the medication tube, and place a thin line of ointment or a few drops of solution along the lower eyelid, preferably without touching the horse's eye. As the horse blinks and closes his eyelids, the medication will coat the entire eye to provide relief and treatment.

Be aware that if you store eye ointment in a warm place, when it is uncapped, a lot of it will come out at once, far more than you'll want. If you keep it in a cold place, on the other hand, it may come out super slowly, making it difficult to apply if the horse won't hold still for very long. Check the ointment's consistency by removing the cap and squeezing just a little to see how much comes out before you begin applying it to a horse's eye.

Serious Eye Damage

If you find that the horse has torn a portion of his eyelid, has a penetrating wound deep into his eye, or has badly damaged the globe of his eyeball, cover the eye with a protective, moist compress bandage until you can obtain professional help.

- Moisten a soft compress with saline before you use it to cover the eye. You can use a Kotex pad, dampened gauze sponges, or a moistened piece of t-shirt for the compress.

- To hold the compress in place, use self-sticking fabric tape like Elastikon®, or stretchable panty hose with ear holes cut out that can be slipped over the horse's face. Secure the stocking with Elastikon® tape.

ALLERGIC REACTIONS

Allergic reactions come in many forms, ranging from skin issues like hives or itching (*urticaria*) to respiratory distress, like equine asthma or anaphylactic shock. The exposure may come from an allergen in the environment or from insect bites.

What to Do For an Acute Allergic Skin Reaction

- Eliminate all food and supplements from the horse's diet other than grass hay.

- Eliminate all medications that are not necessary or required for a horse's ongoing health.

- Stop using fly sprays, as these may cause sensitivity in some horses.

- Switch from pine bedding (or other) to paper bedding. Pine shavings are a common source of skin rashes and hives in horses.

- Don't ride or allow the horse to sweat, as this will worsen his discomfort.

- Wash blankets and grooming equipment, and be sure to rinse out all the soap, which is another potential irritant.

- Monitor the horse's condition—if the condition of his skin isn't steadily improving within 12–24 hours or he is showing signs of respiratory distress, contact a veterinarian for appropriate medical therapy.

Hives

It is common for a horse to suddenly develop hives for no specific reason. Hives are a clinical sign—a reaction the body is having—to proteins (antigens) rather than to a specific disease. A hypersensitivity response to a non-infectious cause or infectious cause is referred to as an *allergy*. Typically, an allergy causes the horse to experience a mild but disagreeable skin reaction, such as hives or itching.

Hives, also referred to as *urticaria*, tend to develop around the neck and shoulders, along the thorax, and across the buttocks. Some refer to these as feed bumps, protein bumps, or heat bumps. Many horses with hives may look bad but are not necessarily uncomfortable or even aware that there is a problem. Hives don't usually affect the general health of the horse, and often disappear within 1–2 days with no treatment necessary.

An allergic reaction on the skin may persist but continuing or worsening signs may lead to a systemic response.

What to Do for Acute Hives

■ Cool water soaks help relieve itching and swelling.

■ Some horses may need treatment with corticosteroids or epinephrine.

- Medications like these only help if they are used for the right kind of allergic reaction. If the horse is experiencing an allergic response because of an infection such as skin parasites, bacteria, or fungus (*ringworm*), even a few days of corticosteroids can turn a mild infection into a severe case that is difficult to resolve. It is always best to figure out the cause of an issue rather than just throwing medication at the problem.

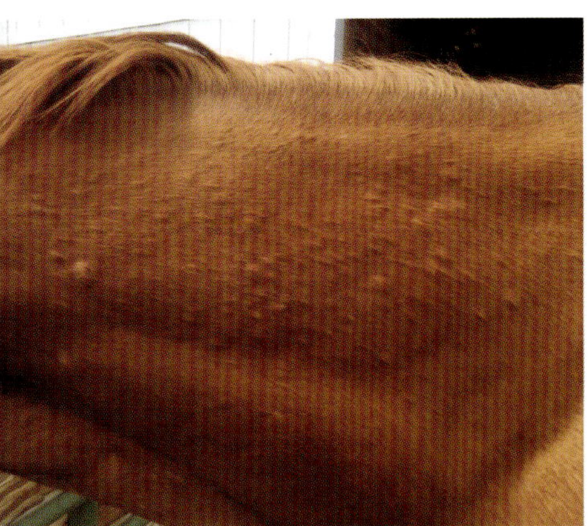

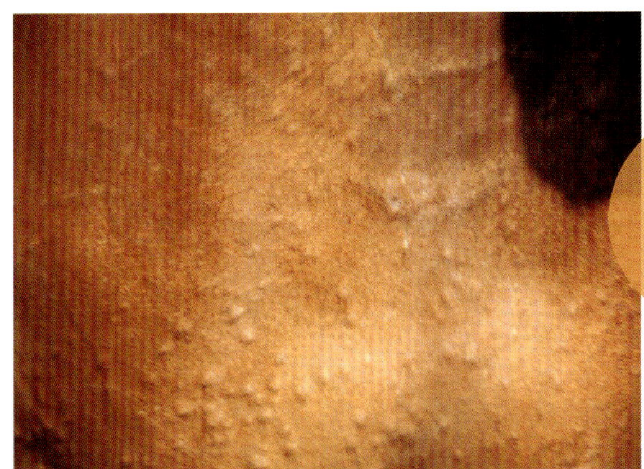

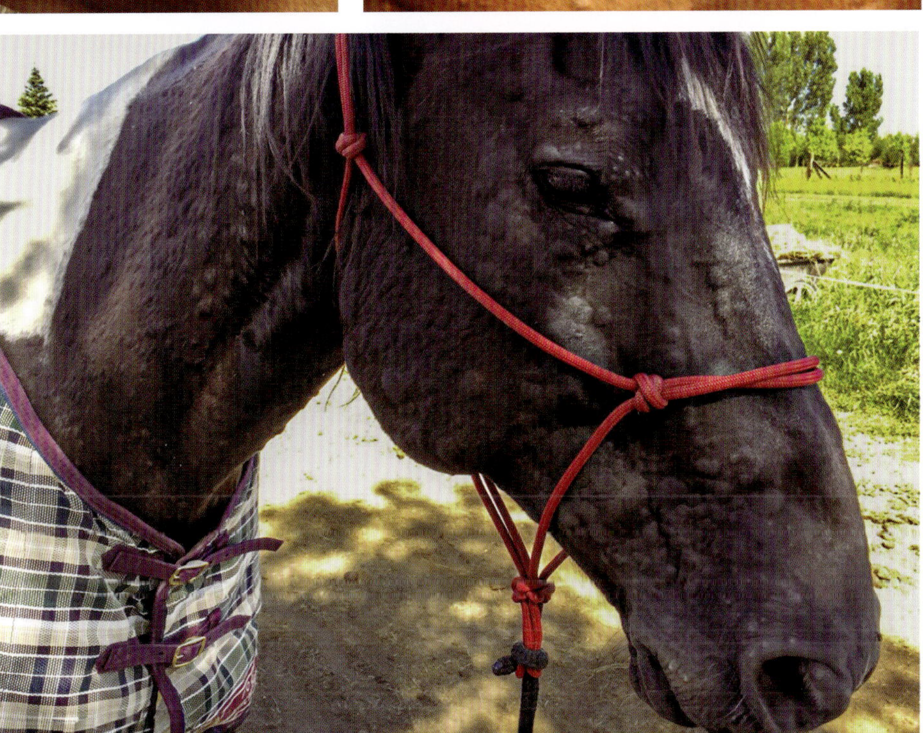

The neck, chest, and buttocks are common locations for an allergic response in the form of hives. Facial swelling with hives is also common.

- Although *antihistamines* don't seem to work very well for acute hives, an antihistamine like *hydroxyzine* may limit an allergic response or work as a preventive, especially for respiratory or skin allergies.

- Refrain from riding a horse, especially in active exercise, if he is experiencing hives. Sweat amplifies physical discomfort around the bumps, and saddle and tack further irritate inflamed tissue.

Angioedema

It is possible for hives to transform into a serious case of *angioedema* and potential *anaphylaxis*. A hive forms as fluid leaks from superficial blood vessels in the skin; the amount of fluid is small due to tissue resistance from the skin over the area. However, with angioedema, internal fluid leaks from deeper vessels and is not contained by tissue pressure, so more fluid escapes. If it develops around a horse's larynx, angioedema can cause a life-threatening situation by pressing on the surrounding tissue enough to narrow the airways or close them entirely. This requires immediate intervention from a veterinarian.

INSECT BITES

Stinging Insects

It is not always possible to avoid even one stinging insect while riding, let alone a swarm; they may also be encountered protecting a nest in proximity to stabled or pastured horses. Wasp or bee stings cause varying levels of discomfort for a horse.

If a horse is stung, especially with multiple stings:

- Stop exercise and keep the horse quiet.

- Give oral Benadryl after consulting a veterinarian for an individualized dose. Typical recommendations are 1–4 milligram/kilogram
(mg/kg) orally.

You can also try some basic home-remedy solutions that vary in their
effectiveness but aren't likely to do harm:

- Cold pack the bite or sting.

- Apply a baking soda-water mixture or calamine lotion to the bite
or sting.

In cases of multiple bites or stings, a horse may need systemic anti-
inflammatory treatment and veterinary intervention.

Spider Bites

Spider bites generally cause a localized reaction in the area of the bite. The horse is
usually sensitive to touch; the surrounding tissue may become inflamed and necrotic,
and hives might develop, with or without itching. Such bites can be managed
following general wound care principles. See the section on wound care below.

WOUNDS AND INJURIES

Evaluation of a Wound

When faced with an acute wound on your horse, inspect it as carefully as possible
to determine whether it is an abrasion, a deeper laceration, or a puncture wound.
Take a photograph for future reference, to track progress, and for comparison in
the event of complications.

- What is the location of the wound? Is it over long bones or a joint, or close to the ground?

- Is the wound superficial or deep?

- Are there structural concerns related to the location?

While a penetrating object can create a "puncture" wound, blunt trauma can also. An impact—like a kick or running into a solid object—can cause tissues to separate, forming an open tract through tissue that looks like a puncture. It can be difficult to determine if a tiny wound or abrasion extends deeper into underlying structures. Unless the answer is clearly obvious, assume a wound has an open tract or pocket in underlying tissue until it is assessed by your veterinarian.

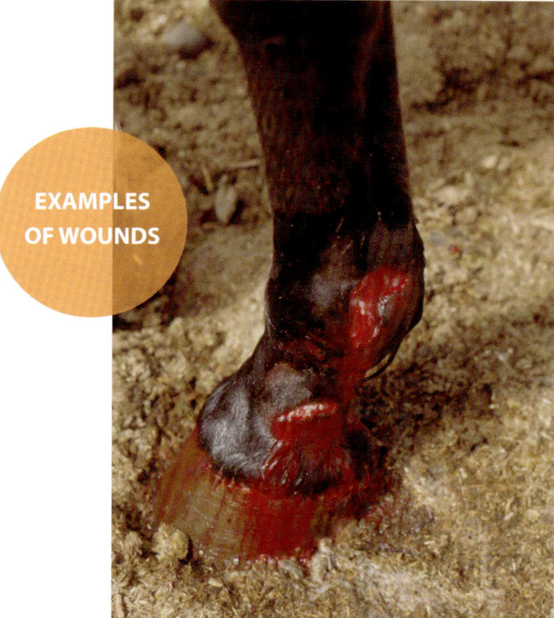
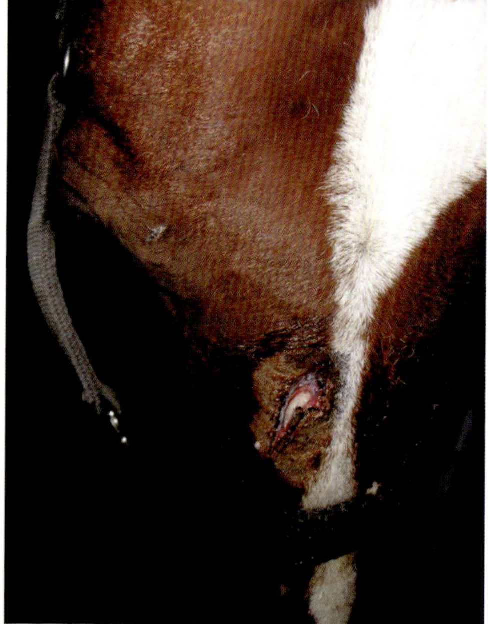

EXAMPLES OF WOUNDS

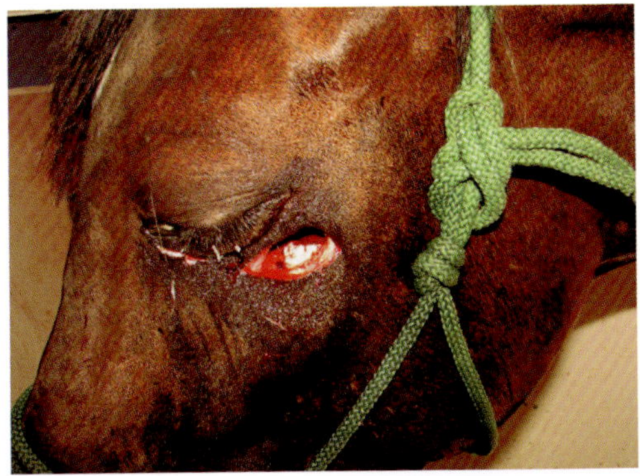

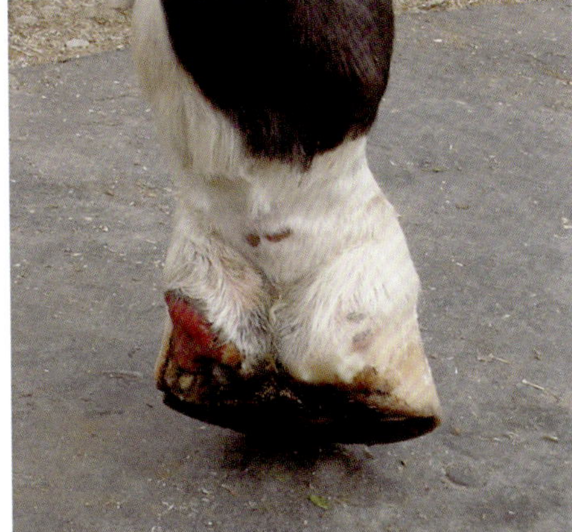

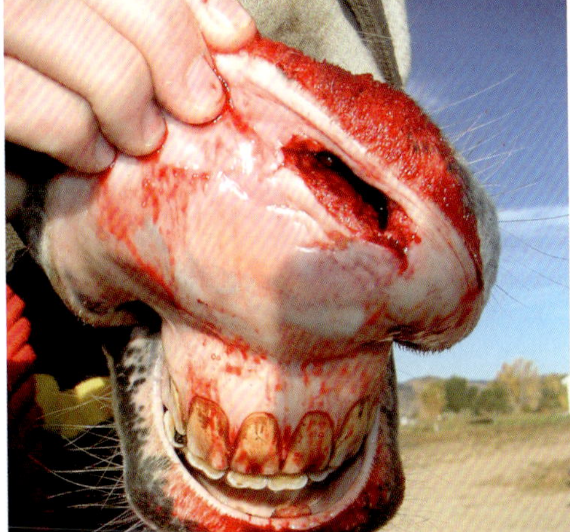

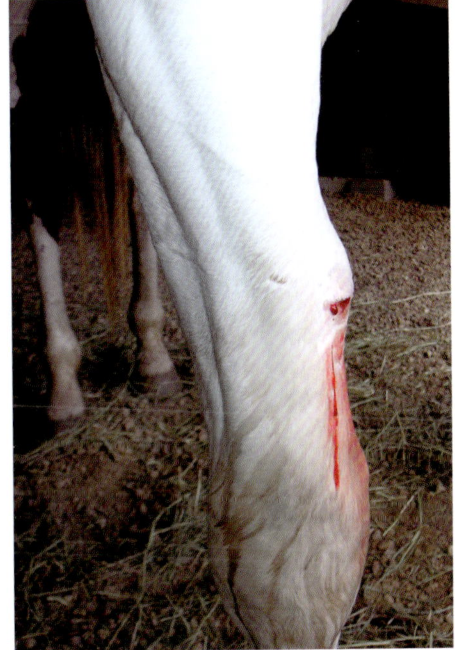

Examples of wounds prior to receiving veterinary care (beginning on facing page and continuing left to right): fetlock, face (exposing bone), below eye (impale wound), heel, lip, forearm (bone swelling and laceration from kick).

EXAMPLES OF WOUNDS

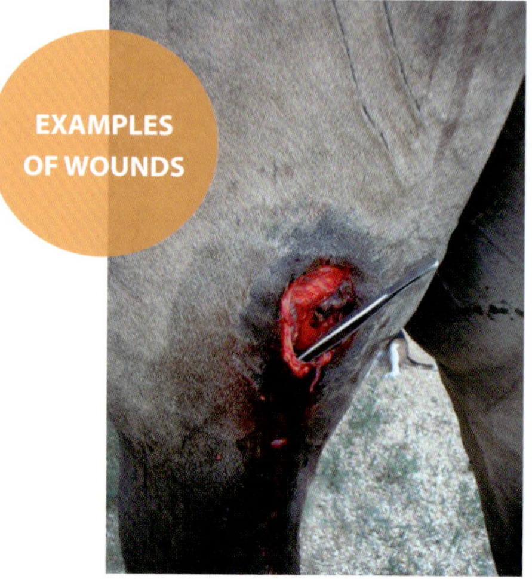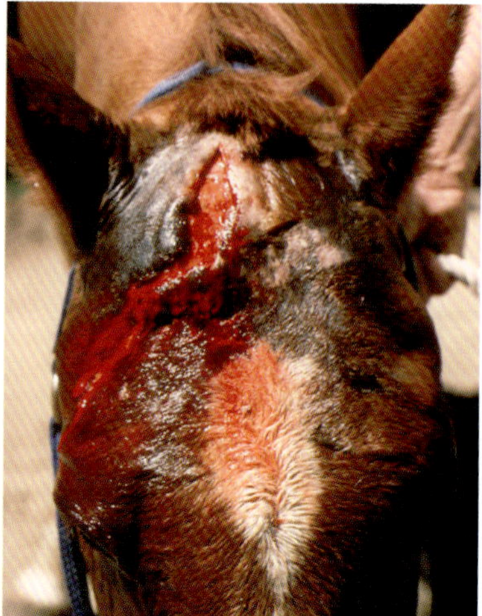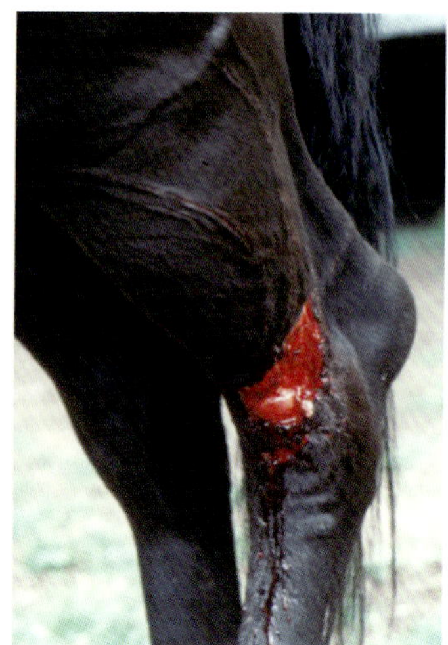

Examples of wounds prior to receiving veterinary care (left to right): thigh (showing pocket in underlying tissue), head, and hock.

Hemorrhage: Active Bleeding

Most wounds on horses tend not to be overly bloody, but a wound involving a vein or artery tends to spurt or ooze blood. Before taking next steps, it is important to first stop the bleeding.

Dealing with Hemorrhage

- Secure a compression bandage snugly around a bleeding wound. Clean bandaging supplies are best, but if they aren't available, form a compress from a ripped portion of cloth or a t-shirt. Apply pressure over the wound using the material and bandage (see p. 105), affixing it with a slight amount of pressure. Or, tape a compress in place or create strips at the ends of the cloth to tie in a knot around the leg.

- If the wound is on the horse's leg, elevate the leg if he'll allow it and encourage the horse to stand quietly.

- Apply ice, when available, over the bandaged wound.

- Firmly press a finger or hand directly onto the bandage over the area of injury and hold it there. Be patient and wait for clotting under the compression bandage.

- Resist the temptation to peek beneath the bandage. Clotting takes at least 12 minutes in most cases, with some large arteries needing as much as 30–60 minutes to clot. Even a little bit of blood—just teaspoons—looks like a lot.

- Check the horse's vital signs. Refer to the section on assessing vital signs (p. 26). Monitor the horse for shock. A horse can lose up to two gallons of blood before suffering a life-threatening cardiovascular crisis and shock. Refer to the section on dehydration and shock (p. 69).

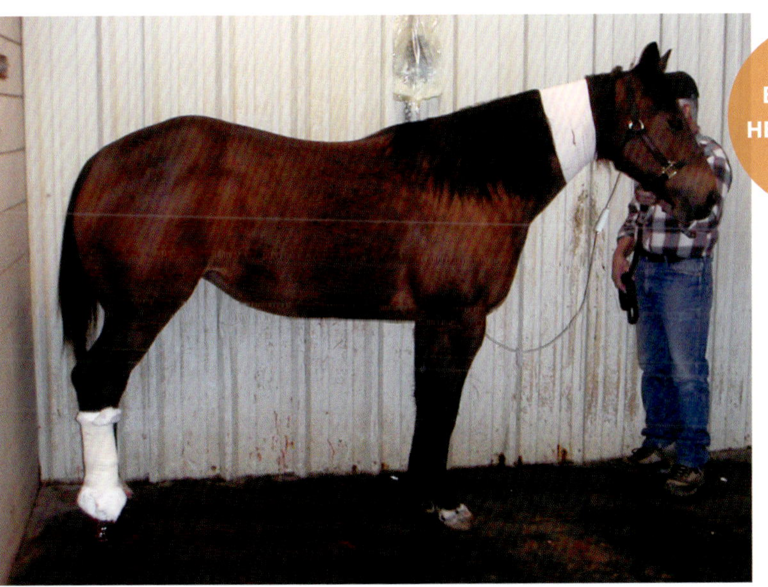

Hemorrhage (hind leg) with a compression bandage and obvious blood loss necessitating IV fluid replacement.

With a wound to the leg, if bleeding won't stop with direct bandaging, it may be appropriate to apply a temporary tourniquet snugly around the leg, above the wound.

- Use a piece of latigo from a saddle, a leather throatlatch, or a shoelace to make a tourniquet. Don't leave the tourniquet in place for more than 10–15 minutes; otherwise, there is a risk of tendon and circulatory damage. It may be best to pad the tendon over which the tourniquet is placed. Confer with your veterinarian whenever possible.

Cleaning a Wound

The objective in wound care is to manage each stage of wound treatment in a way that enables the wound to heal as quickly as possible. You cannot speed up healing but it can be slowed by inappropriate handling of a wound. An optimal healing environment relies on following hygienic wound care procedures.

- Provided there is no hemorrhage that needs rapid compression bandaging, remove as much debris and contamination as you can from a wound as soon as possible.

- If the horse is cooperative and allows you to safely handle the area around a wound, trim or shave away overlying and surrounding hair before you begin cleaning it. Be sure to remove remnants of hair from the wound, which could cause irritation the same way a foreign body would.

- If your horse won't allow safe handling of the area near the wound, try to spray it—from a safe distance—with water from a garden hose to remove debris and contamination.

For cleaning the wound itself, use saline solution if you have it, or make a salt solution by adding ½ tablespoon of table salt per quart of distilled water. Any degree of cleaning is helpful, even if just using tap water; that is better than not cleaning the wound at all.

Prepare an antiseptic solution by adding one of the following solutions to distilled or clean salt water (or tap water, if that's all you have). Dilute antiseptic solutions, since full-strength concentrations are toxic to the tissues you're trying to treat.

- "Tamed iodine" (dilute or povidone-iodine) solution, mixed at 10 milliliters (ml) per quart of saline water—this concentration approximates the color of weak tea.

- Chlorhexidine solution, mixed at 15–25 ml per quart of saline water.

Next steps:

- Scrub the wound with either tamed povidone-iodine (Betadine) or chlorhexidine scrub soap for 10 minutes. Soak sterile gauze sponges in antiseptic solution, apply the scrub soap, and clean. To avoid recontamination of the wound, discard soiled gauze frequently and use fresh pieces.

- Once the wound is cleaned, rinse it well with saline water-antiseptic solution to remove all scrub soap that could be an irritant to healing.

- Allow the wound to air dry, and then apply a *water-soluble* topical antibiotic ointment or cream. Examples of water-soluble wound salves include triple antibiotic ointment, chlorhexidine cream, and silver sulfadiazine cream.

■ Or cover the wound with a mixture of povidone-iodine (Betadine) and sugar, referred to as "sugardine." The osmotic action of sugar pulls moisture and swelling from the wound and provides anti-bacterial effects.

What *Not* to Do for Wounds

Above all, when managing a wound, you want to "do no harm." With that in mind, there are several things you want to avoid.

■ If you think a wound has the potential to be sutured, don't apply anything to it prior to bandaging, except a *water-soluble* cream or ointment that easily washes away. A petroleum-based ointment interferes with healing on a wound that needs sutures and may cause stitches to come apart. You can use petroleum-based ointments below a wound to help prevent skin scald from leaking fluids running downward.

■ Don't apply sprays or caustic chemicals to an open wound. Spray medications dry out the edges of a wound, leaving less tissue available to pull together with stitches. Dry tissue loses its blood supply, and needs to be cut away to expose fresh, bleeding tissue before healing can proceed. A need to trim away tissue is likely to increase tension on the wound's edges when it's sutured, or may result in a longer healing time if it must heal by second intention with granulation tissue.

■ Caustic chemicals are irritating and toxic to tissue, and may cause a horse to react violently if applied to a wound. These include:

• Hydrogen peroxide—this is only useful for cleaning blood off the leg, away from a wound.

- Alcohol.

- Full strength (7 percent) tincture of iodine.

Tetanus Prophylaxis

Check your horse's tetanus status and ensure that his most recent immunization was within the last year. If there is any question about this, have your veterinarian give him a booster using tetanus toxoid.

Bandaging a Wound

A bandage fulfills multiple functions and provides: a) protection from contamination and insects; b) tissue support; c) stability; and d) warmth. Keeping a wound clean is a main ingredient for successful healing.

Bandaging materials you'll want to have in your first aid supply box include:

- A non-stick sterile pad (Telfa®) to apply directly over the wound once cleaned. Antibiotic ointment can be applied to this non-stick pad.

- Cotton (sheet or roll type) or Combine ABD pad to wrap around the area of the leg to bandage. This cushions against uneven bandage pressure. Position this with no wrinkles.

- A roll of gauze to hold the cotton in place, if needed.

- Elastic, self-stick fabric bandaging material such as Elastikon® or Elastoplast.

- Gorilla tape, duct tape, or adhesive tape to secure the ends of the Elastikon® bandage.

The procedure for applying a bandage varies depending on the materials you are comfortable using, but here is a standard technique for applying a successful bandage. Once the area is dry:

- Apply water-soluble, antibiotic ointment or cream to the wound or on a non-stick (Telfa®) pad.

- Cover the wound with a non-stick (Telfa®) pad.

- Or use a wet-to-dry bandage—lightly soak gauze with diluted antiseptic solution and place it directly on the wound.

- Follow this by wrapping the limb using padding such as a layer of roll cotton, Combine ABD pad, sanitary pad, or leg quilt. Make sure there are no wrinkles. Pad well over bony prominences—for example, the

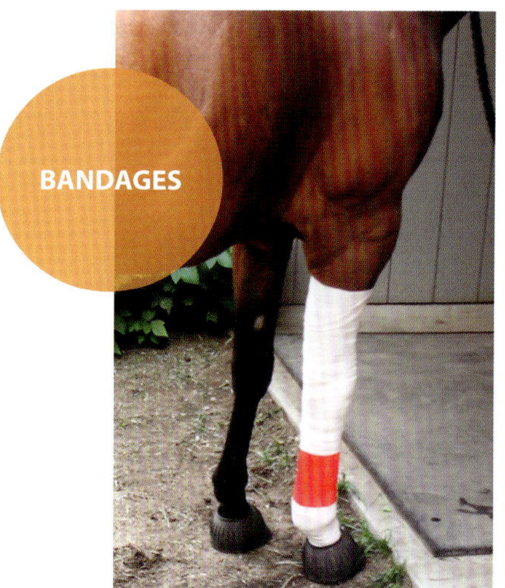
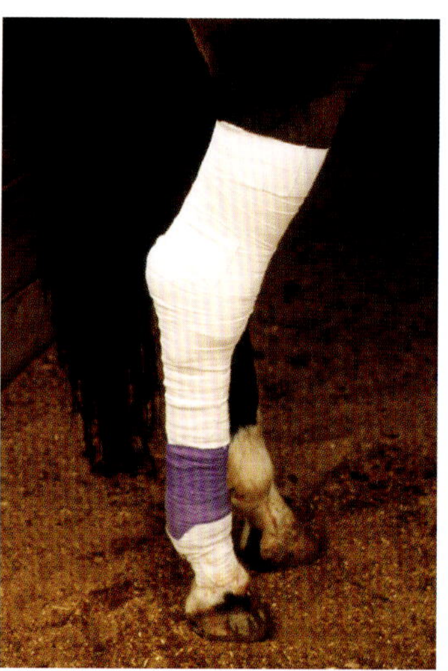
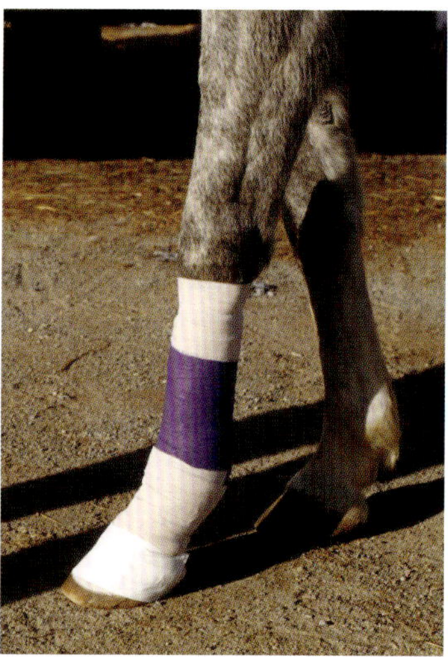

BANDAGES

Examples of bandaging (from left to right, including facing page): front leg, hind leg, compression, front leg with boot (to keep heel wrap from sliding up), hoof (no boot), and head (for impale wound near the eye).

sesamoid bones of the fetlock, carpal accessory bone on the back
of the knee, and point of the hock—to avoid pressure damage to
the skin.

- Optional: Wrap gauze around the padding to hold it in place,
especially if you don't have an assistant.

- Prepare to apply the outer layer of self-stick bandaging material.
Elastikon® is the safest material to use, since it doesn't tend to bind
tightly like VetWrap® or Co-Flex do. Elastikon® has more give and
flexibility than other wrapping materials, so it is the best choice to
avoid restricting blood circulation or binding tendons. Apply this
outer material with light compression—it should be snug but not so
tight that it restricts circulation.

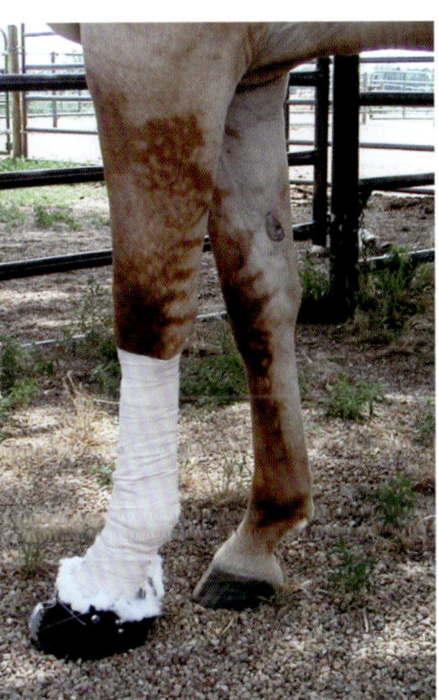
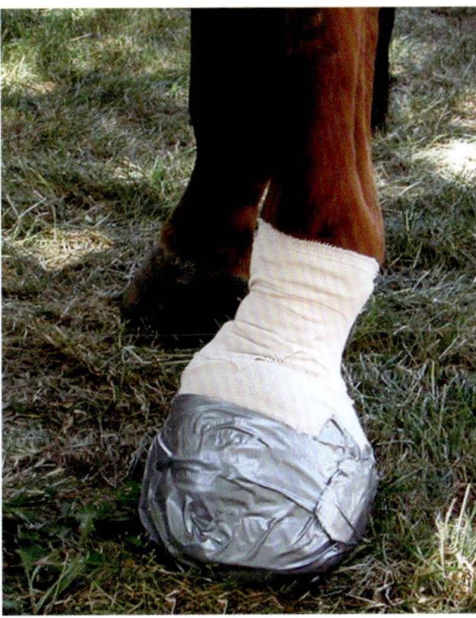
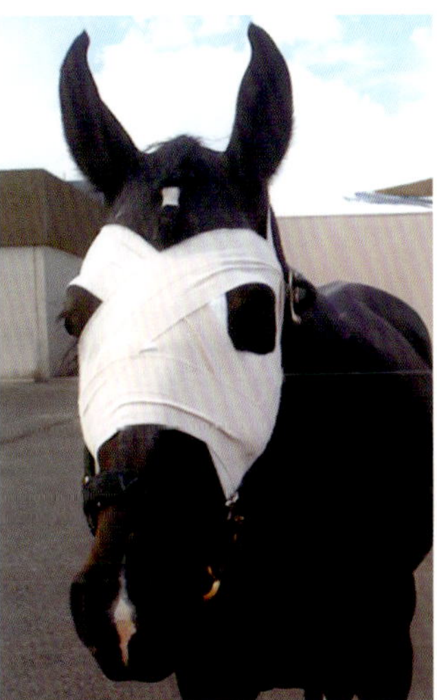

- In the middle of each roll of Elastikon® is a visible red line that serves as a guide to show you where to overlap the bandage with each wrap around the leg. Just barely cover that red line with each turn. That keeps the bandage from slipping apart. Spiral the bandage as you wrap the leg to further secure it in place on hair not covered with padding.

- As you unroll the bandage material to wrap the leg, pull when the material is over the front of the limb, and then lay the material across the back of the limb without tightening over the rear of the leg. This is important to prevent inadvertent tightening and constriction of the rear tendons or blood supply.

- Once the self-stick bandage roll is applied, add a couple of small strips of Gorilla or duct or adhesive tape to secure the very end of the Elastikon® roll so it doesn't peel up and begin to unravel. These kinds of tape have no stretch or breathability, so they should *not* be wrapped all the way around the leg, as they will restrict circulation. Apply as strips that don't encircle the leg but are there to hold down the ends of the Elastikon®.

Change a bandage every 2–3 days (or as often as your veterinarian recommends) to remove contamination, moisture, and sloughing tissue.

Bandaging of High or Low Wounds

For wounds higher up on the leg—from the knee or hock and up—use a "stacking" procedure to prevent slippage. First, place a full bandage starting at the top of the cannon bone to incorporate the fetlock below. Then, apply a carpal or hock bandage over the wound and connect it directly to the cannon bandage while also securing it at the top of the leg (forearm or gaskin) with elastic tape. The cannon bandage keeps the carpal or hock bandage from slipping down.

For a bandage placed low down near the foot, incorporate the heel bulb and upper hoof with Elastikon®. To prevent slippage, make a figure eight with the bandage around the heel bulbs. This prevents it from riding up onto the pastern.

For hoof or pastern wounds, once the area is bandaged, place a hoof boot on the foot to hold the bandage in place. Before placing the boot, apply cotton over the bottom of the foot and up the sides to keep debris out of the boot.

HEMATOMA/SEROMA AND FIRM SWELLINGS

An impact trauma like a kick or a fall can cause swelling beneath the skin, and even beneath subcutaneous tissue. Sometimes, a muscle belly is torn by the impact. If there is bleeding, this is called a *hematoma*; if the swelling is filled with yellow or blood-tinged serum, it is called a *seroma*. Swelling may form a lump as small as a golf ball or as large as grapefruit in size, or larger.

When you push on this kind of swelling with your finger, it feels like a water balloon, with fluid bouncing in waves beneath your finger.

What to Do for a Fluid-Filled Swelling

Usually, these situations are *not* urgent emergencies; it is typically best to wait a few days before draining a swelling, especially in a torn muscle belly. Pressure from the fluid within the swelling will limit the amount of blood or serum that seeps into the area.

In the meantime:

- Apply cold therapy—an ice pack—to slow bleeding and limit swelling. Refer to the section on cryotherapy (p. 126).

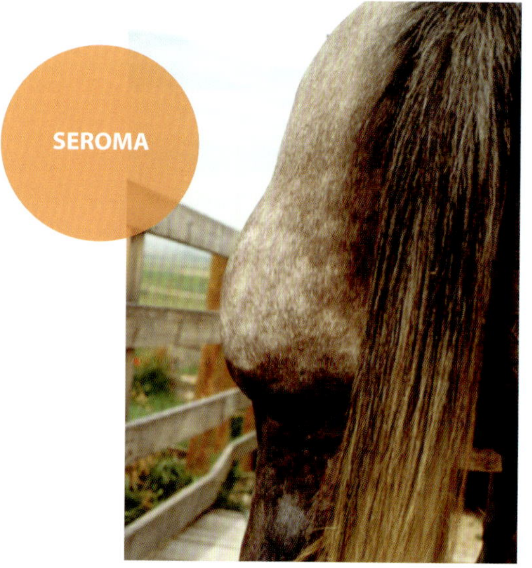

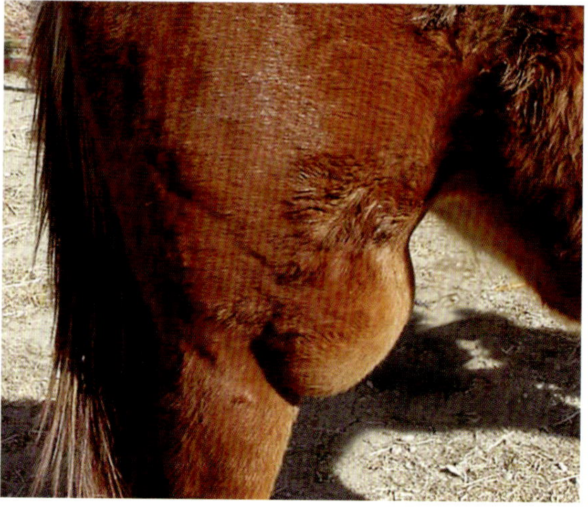

Examples of a seroma.

- Keep the horse confined for several days to limit his movement so he doesn't develop additional muscle and fascial trauma that could stimulate more bleeding or seepage.

Firm Swelling in Odd Places: "Pigeon Breast"

In some parts of the country, there are cycles of a syndrome referred to as "pigeon breast" or "pigeon fever," caused by the bacteria *Corynebacterium pseudotuberculosis*. A horse is inoculated with the bacteria through biting flies. An abscess forms with fluid that is thick, creamy, and non-odorous. These abscesses must be drained and flushed, with all materials disposed of properly to avoid fly access or ground contamination.

With this condition, swelling occurs most often on the chest—hence the moniker "pigeon breast"—but can also develop around the groin, prepuce, or udder, or in other odd places, including positions where it blocks lymphatic drainage and causes leg swelling. In rare cases, a horse will develop internal abscessation, which is challenging to treat.

SNAKEBITE

Whether you are living and riding in the desert country or prairies of the American West, or in the woods of the East or South, it's good to be on the lookout for snakes. Rattlesnakes are common throughout the United States, while cottonmouths (aka water moccasins) and copperheads are most abundant in the southern areas of the country. These are the species a horse is most likely to encounter. Poisonous snakes have elliptical pupils in their eyes; the pupils of non-poisonous snakes are round.

Most snakes are timid, and a horse's hooves shake the ground enough to send a snake on its way most of the time—unless, of course, the horse steps on him or comes into close contact. Or, as happens most commonly, a horse browsing grass may inadvertently bump his nose close to a resting snake.

Unlike dogs or people, in most cases horses do not succumb rapidly to the effects of snake venom. In fact, many snakebites are "dry," meaning no venom is injected. Usually, the bigger problem is the injection of *Clostridial sp.* bacteria into the wounds, and the risk of anaerobic infection. Another concern with a snake strike is the rapid swelling that accompanies the bite; if the horse is bitten on the face, this swelling could obscure the airways and make breathing difficult. And, in some cases, effects on the liver from a snakebite can cause a horse to be photosensitive if he is out in direct sun.

■ Generally, you'll have plenty of time to get your horse to veterinary help. In the meantime, you can try a few things:

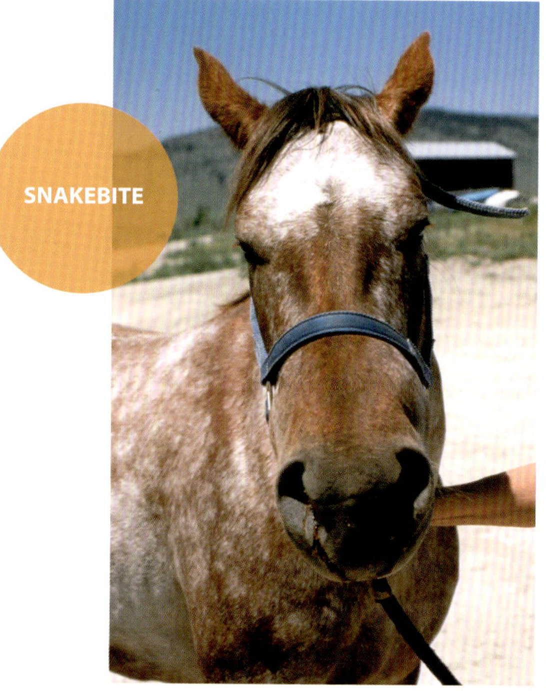
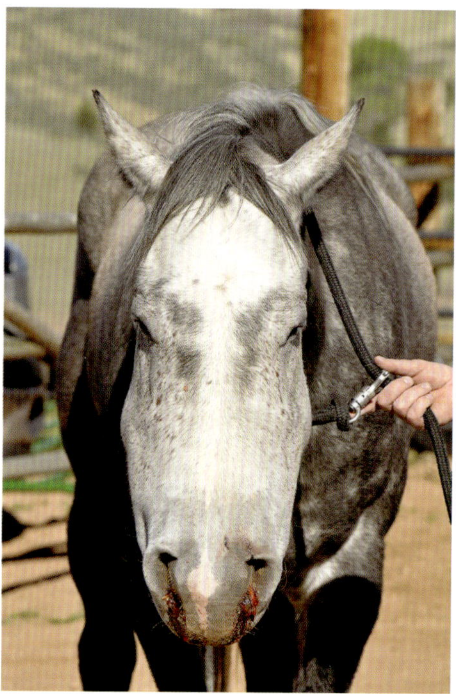

Head swelling often accompanies a snakebite to the face.

- Keep your horse as quiet and calm as possible to slow his heart rate; this also slows the circulation of venom through his body.

- Obtain veterinary help as soon as possible for appropriate treatment, which may include intravenous fluids and antivenin.

- Once you are back at the barn, stable the horse out of the sun.

- If you have antibiotics in your emergency kit, start the horse on a dose of a broad-spectrum antibiotic to forestall infection. It is best to confer with your veterinarian first.

■ A dose of an NSAID, like phenylbutazone or Banamine®, helps control inflammation, pain, and swelling to some degree. Discuss with your veterinarian before administering.

■ If the horse experiences facial swelling that interferes with his breathing, then cut two pieces of garden hose into 6–8-inch sections, lubricate them with cooking oil, and slide them as far into both nostrils as possible, leaving about an inch protruding from the nostrils. Secure them with Elastikon® tape. Swelling associated with a snakebite generally affects the external tissues of the muzzle rather than the inner portions of the airways or throat so the tubes help keep the airways open.

■ Update tetanus prophylaxis as needed.

What Not to Do

■ If the wound is on a limb, do not apply a tourniquet.

■ Do not try to cut the tissue over the fang marks as this might cause more tissue damage and the horse could react violently.

■ Do not try to "suck out" the venom with your mouth.

■ Do not apply hot or cold packs as this can cause more damage.

Currently there is a commercial vaccine (Red Rock Biologics) available for rattlesnake bite in horses as a preventive measure for horses living in high-risk areas.

POISONING

There are a number of toxic materials that a horse might ingest. When faced with a sick horse emergency where it is difficult to discern the cause, consider a potential poisoning, especially at certain times of year when toxic plants might be abundant in pasture or as ornamentals around the property.

Besides contacting your veterinarian, another resource you can reach out to for advice is a local or regional university or equine referral hospital. You can also call poison hotline resources. These are primarily set up for small animal incidents, but some may be able to provide help with poisoning in horses:

- American Society for the Prevention of Cruelty to Animals (ASCPA) Poison Helpline: (888) 426-4435.

- Animal Poison Control Center (APCC): (855) 764-7661.

- National Animal Poison Control Center (NAPPC) at the University of Illinois: (900) 680-0000 or (800) 548-2423.

There may be a fee for using these hotlines, but they are available 24/7.

Plants

Plants are one of the main culprits in horse poisonings. The list is not exhaustive, but here are some common ones (in alphabetical order) that a horse might encounter that could cause an emergency situation:

- *Alkaloid toxicosis*—caused by a variety of plants, including:

  - Locoweed (*Astragalus* and *Oxytropis spp.*) can cause alkaloid toxicity—neurologic damage, emaciation, weakness and loss of muscular control, dull hair coat, depression, reproductive dysfunction and abortion, and congestive heart failure.

- Lupine leads to reproductive failure and fetal abnormalities.

- Poison hemlock—affects the central nervous system, causing symptoms such as uncoordinated movement, muscle tremors, paralysis, frequent urination, difficulty breathing, and collapse.

■ Alsike clover—liver failure, jaundice, abdominal pain, photosensitivity, skin sloughing.

■ Black locust trees—abdominal pain/gastritis, diarrhea, fecal blood, lameness, dilated pupils, weakness, depression, death.

■ Black walnut as bedding—laminitis, edema, colic.

■ Blue-green algae in stagnant water—colic, muscle tremors, diarrhea, yellow gums, and seizures.

■ Boxelder maple seeds hypoglycin A toxin—tremors, weakness, stiffness, dark urine, rapid breathing, death.

■ Bracken fern inhibits absorption of vitamin B1 (thiamine)—this can cause weight loss, weakness, gait abnormalities, muscle twitching, abnormal heart rate and rhythm, inability to rise, and death. Horsetail causes similar symptoms due to an enzyme that destroys thiamine.

■ Buttercup—irritated mouth and throat tissues, colic, diarrhea.

■ Cocklebur leaves—rapid and weak pulse, labored breathing, spasms of leg and neck muscles.

- Cyanide from specific plants like chokecherries—difficulty breathing, red gums, incoordination, staggering, seizures, collapse, death.

- Hoary alyssum (mustard family) is toxic when more than one-third of the forage consumed is this plant. Signs—leg swelling, fever, stiff joints, reluctance to move, diarrhea, intravascular hemolysis and shock, laminitis.

- Lantana (yellow or red sage)—jaundice, skin sloughing, photosensitization, respiratory distress, diarrhea, and low blood sugar and weakness.

- Milkweed—weakness, respiratory difficulties, cardiotoxicity, colic, diarrhea, muscle tremors, seizures, head pressing, coma, death.

- Nightshade family—jimsonweed, horse nettle, potato and tomato plants and skins, and deadly nightshade lead to central nervous system effects such as dilated pupils, trembling, paralysis, shock, coma, muscle tremors, incoordination, and gastrointestinal signs of abdominal pain, diarrhea, or impaction.

- Oak trees with gallotannin toxin—poor appetite, weight loss, bloody urine and black tarry diarrhea; increased drinking and urination, dehydration, kidney failure, edema, colic, and death.

- Oleander is a cardiotoxic plant—abdominal pain, colic, muscle tremors, labored breathing, ataxia, weak pulse, irregular heartbeats, diarrhea, seizures, collapse, sudden death.

- Red maple, especially wilting or fallen autumn leaves, destroys red blood cells—breathing difficulties, jaundice, colic, bloody or brown urine, fever, death.

- Rhododendron—stomach irritation, abdominal pain, abnormal heart rate and rhythm, convulsions, coma, death.

- Water hemlock—central nervous system effects like nervousness, breathing difficulties, muscle tremors, collapse, convulsions, death.

- White snakeroot containing tremetol—trembling, stiffness, ataxia, damage to liver and heart muscle and heart failure, coma, death.

- Yellow star thistle—difficulty eating and swallowing, lethargy, neurologic signs such as twitching lips, flicking tongue, involuntary chewing, drowsiness, difficulty grasping or chewing food, head pressing, weakness, circling, wandering. Russian knapweed induces similar problems due to brain damage.

- Yew trees—muscle trembling, incoordination, colic, slow heart rate, death.

Molds and Fungi

- *Aflatoxicosis*—liver damage, excessive bleeding, muscle tremors, incoordination, yellow gums or skin.

- Moldy sweet clover—hemorrhage, bruising, red spotted gums, nosebleeds, stiffness and lameness.

- Moldy sweet corn contaminated with *fumonisin*—*equine leukoencephalomalacia* or liver damage with yellow gums, incoordination, blindness, circling, recumbency, and sudden death.

- Ryegrass staggers—muscle tremors, incoordination, recumbency.
- Slaframine black patch fungal toxin in legumes—diarrhea, mild abdominal pain, salivation.

- Tall fescue grass contaminated with toxic endophyte fungus, especially ergovaline—prolonged gestation, decreased milk production, abortion, stillbirth, dystocia.

Minerals and Micronutrients in Excess or in a Deficit

- Heavy metals such as lead, arsenic, mercury—colic, seizures, incoordination, recumbency, organ failure and death.

- Iron from supplements, water, grass, or hay—jaundice, rough hair coat, weight loss, head pressing.

- Nitrate and nitrite found in contaminated forage or water, especially in the presence of fertilizer—brown blood disease from reduced oxygen transport in the body leading to weakness, tremors, recumbency, blue gums, and sudden death.

- Oxalates from plants that bind calcium—lameness, bone fractures, increased urination, change in head shape.

- Selenium—lethargy, abdominal pain, death, or more acute forms include cracking or sloughing of the hoof wall, lameness, hair loss.

Insecticides and Dewormers

- Organophosphates—hyperexcitability, colic, muscle tremors, patchy sweat, salivation, diarrhea, stiff-legged gait or staggering, collapse, respiratory failure.

- Carbamates—similar signs as organophosphates.

Poison Animal Baits

- Containing strychnine, arsenic, or zinc, for example—hyperexcitability, tremors, seizures, respiratory depression, collapse, death.

ACUTE LAMENESS

Character of a Lameness

A true musculoskeletal emergency is one in which a horse suddenly appears very lame and is reluctant to put significant weight on the limb.

Begin by looking for a simple problem, like a stone, pebble, or piece of wood that is wedged in the clefts of the frog. Look for thorns, cactus spines, or goat head stickers that may have lodged in the tender, soft tissues of the heel bulbs, coronary band, or frog clefts. Look for a nail in any portion of the foot.

Check the digital pulses behind each fetlock (see photo on p. 27). A bounding pulse typically indicates significant inflammation in the lower limb.

Classifying the Lameness by Grade

The American Association of Equine Practitioners (AAEP) has developed a grading system to classify the degree of lameness a horse is experiencing. An acute lameness emergency usually is described as Grade 4 or 5 on this scale of 0–5:

- **Grade 0**: Lameness is not perceptible under any circumstances.

- **Grade 1**: Lameness is difficult to observe and is not consistently apparent, regardless of circumstances, such as the horse moving under saddle, on circles, on inclines, or on a hard surface.

- **Grade 2**: Lameness is difficult to observe at a walk or when trotting in a straight line, but is consistently apparent under certain circumstances, such as carrying weight (of a rider), circling, inclines, or hard surfaces, as examples.

- **Grade 3**: Lameness is consistently observable at a trot under all circumstances, including on a straight line.

- **Grade 4**: Lameness is obvious at a walk.

- **Grade 5**: Lameness produces minimal weight bearing in motion and/or at rest, or a complete inability to move.

The higher the lameness score, the worse the lameness. It is best to stop riding a horse with any level of lameness until the source and reason can be identified, so as not to worsen an injury.

Mild to Moderate Lameness: Grades 1, 2, 3

Grades 1, 2, and 3 describe a horse that is still able to put weight on the limb and can trot when asked.

Significant Weight-Bearing Lameness: Grade 4

Grade 4 lameness means that the horse is quite lame; he still might touch his toe to the ground for support but without putting his full weight on the limb. This degree of lameness is apparent at the walk and on turns.

Causes of Grade 4 lameness can include:

- A foot abscess.

- Acute joint injury.

- Progressive degenerative arthritis.

- A ligament or tendon injury or tear.

- A chip fracture in a joint.

- Laminitis.

Severe Non-Weight-Bearing Lameness: Grade 5

A horse with Grade 5 lameness refuses to put any weight on his leg no matter what. When asked to move, he will hold the injured leg off the ground and hop on the opposite limb. This is referred to as being "three-legged lame."

Such an injury is serious and a true emergency situation. The horse may have:

- A foot abscess or deep hoof nail puncture.

- A bone fracture.

- A joint or tendon sheath penetration, infection, or both.

- Serious soft tissue injury, such as with a ligament or tendon tear.

■ *Cellulitis*, which is a diffuse bacterial infection of the skin and subcutaneous tissues that spreads extensively through tissue planes. Sometimes there is an obvious wound that has allowed bacteria to enter the body, but other times, there is no obvious entry point for the infection. Impact trauma or micro-abrasions from leg boots are examples of potential causes for cellulitis that don't involve a wound. Damaged tissue can still be infected with bacteria from the bloodstream (*hematogenous* spread). It is reported that 50 percent of cellulitis cases are caused by infection with *Staphylococcal* or *Streptococcal* bacterial species.

CELLULITIS

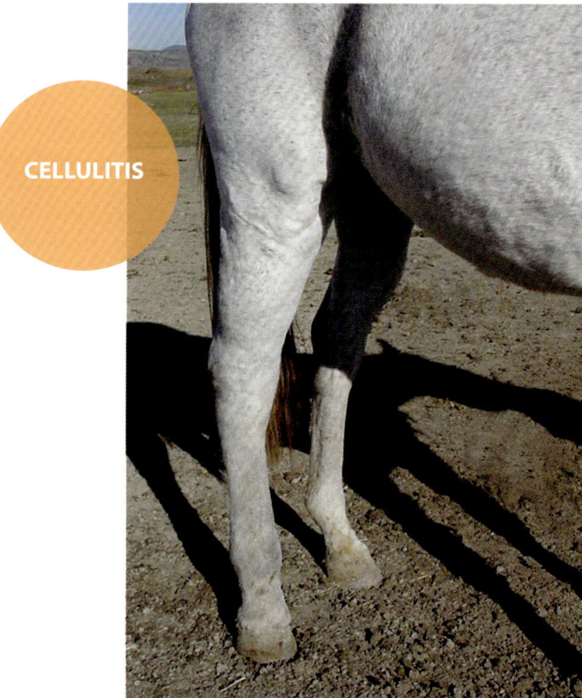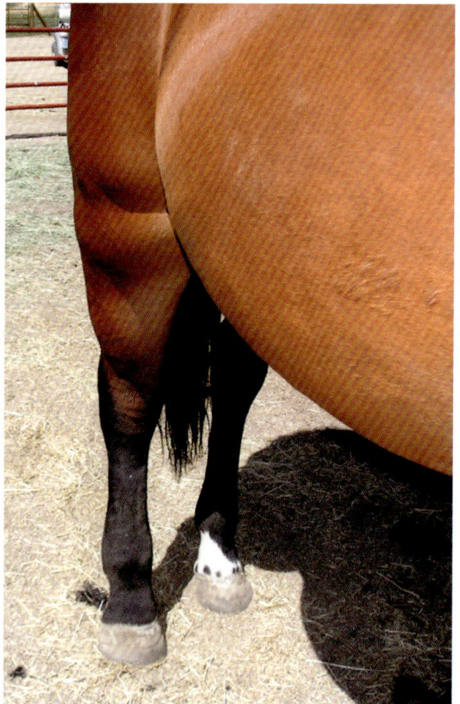

Examples of cellulitis in the right hind limb.

What to Look For

Is There Swelling?

Observe the horse closely when he is standing still and then moving:

- Does the horse appear comfortable, or is he showing stiffness or lameness?

- Is only one leg swollen, or more than one?

Are There Other Abnormalities?

Feel the affected limb(s) and note any abnormalities:

- Is there heat in the limb?

- Does the horse pull away due to pain following a light touch or firmer palpation of the swollen area?

- Do you feel irregularities in the skin or hair such as scabs and crusts, moist or oozing discharge, or abnormal lumps?

- Does the skin crackle when touched due to air trapped beneath the tissues, or due to a rampant anaerobic bacterial infection? This is a potentially life-threatening situation that requires immediate veterinary attention.

- How lame is the horse, and to what degree? Refer to the AAEP Lameness Scale in the section on classifying lameness (p. 120).

- Do you see or feel any drainage or signs of a puncture or wound?

- Is the swelling in proximity to or within a synovial structure, like a joint, bursa, or tendon sheath?

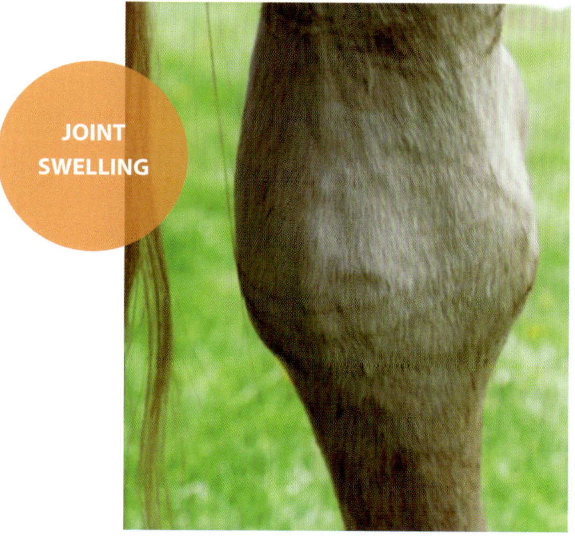

Joint swelling at the hock.

- Is the swelling localized to a specific area, or is there generalized pitting edema? (*Pitting edema* refers to pitting or dimpling of swollen tissue after being pressed on with a finger; the indented tissue does not recover its smooth contours.)

- Does the horse have a fever that is possibly indicative of a systemic problem, like a viral or bacterial infection? Isolate the horse and refer to the section on biosecurity (p. 154).

With obvious swelling of a limb, you may be able to locate an injury, especially by comparing each leg to its opposite. Not all lameness problems are accompanied by swelling, particularly with a hoof injury.

Keep in mind that swelling higher in the limb often diffuses downward from gravity, meaning the lower limb may be swollen because it's beneath the injury and not because it is a problem in the lower limb itself. Diffuse swelling makes it more difficult to determine the exact location of an injury.

If you identify swelling:

- Look carefully for a wound—it could be an abrasion or a puncture wound that is difficult to see. Apply appropriate wound care as described in the section on wound care (p. 97).

- Ice pack or cold hose the area for 15–20 minutes at a time, 2–3 times per day. Refer to the section on cryotherapy and icing (p. 126).

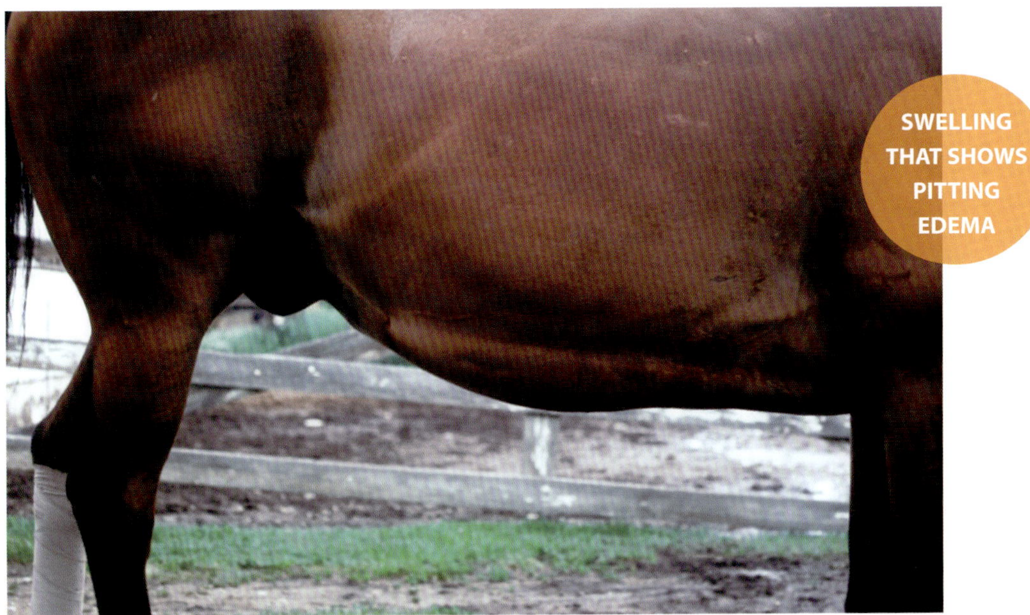

When you push your finger into a swelling like this abdominal swelling, the "pit" or "dimple" remains due to fluid accumulation in the tissues, which is called *pitting edema*.

■ Apply a compression bandage to the lower limb. This helps contain swelling in a lower limb injury, and also helps to prevent diffusing gravitational swelling from an injury higher on the leg. Reapply this bandage following each cold therapy application. Refer to the section on applying bandages (p. 105).

■ Confine the horse until your veterinarian can assess the seriousness of the injury.

■ Administer an NSAID under the advisement of a veterinarian.

Cryotherapy and Icing

With inflammation comes an increase in blood vessel permeability, and that brings more tissue "fluid" to the area, which causes even more swelling. The use of cryotherapy (icing) is instrumental in:

- Slowing circulation to help reduce swelling and pain.

- Decreasing metabolic needs of the tissue.

- Decreasing inflammatory mediators that cause inflammation to persist. (Inflammatory mediators are molecules and proteins that are produced by cells in response to injury or infection, and that play a key role in an immune response.)

- Providing a local anesthetic effect to reduce pain.

All these benefits provide comfort to a horse.

"Cold today and hot tamale" is a simple reminder of how to approach managing inflammation. Cold "today" may be appropriate not just for one day, but instead for several days to weeks, depending on the severity of an injury. Icing addresses some of the physical signs of inflammation but won't completely stop the inflammatory process, which does have a role in assisting healing. With an open wound, icing directly on the wound is not recommended because of exposed and open tissues.

Icing Tips

- The target temperature with cryotherapy is 50 degrees Fahrenheit. This *cannot* be achieved with cold tap water and a hose. It requires the use of ice, ice boots, or cold water and ice immersion.

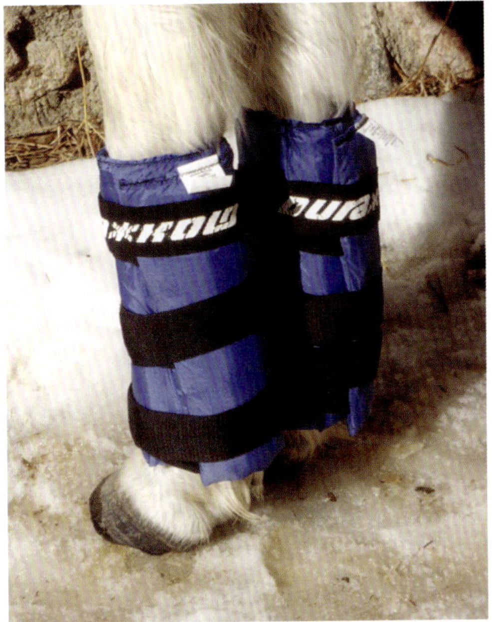

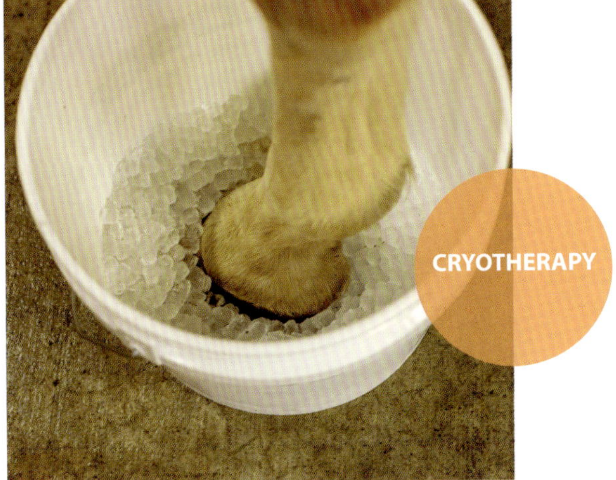

Effective cryotherapy can be achieved with ice boots or immersion in an ice water bath of ice (shown above) mixed with cold water.

- Do not apply ice directly to a horse's skin. Wrap ice in a thin, damp cloth to avoid skin "burn." Then it is safe to apply to the horse.

- Wet the horse's hair down to the skin before placing commercial ice boots. This eliminates insulating effects from the hair and makes it easier for cold to reach underlying tissues.

- Ice for no more than 20–30 minutes at a time, and then remove the ice to restore circulation. Ice frequently for short periods and allow intervals with no ice in between, rather than leaving ice in place for extended periods. Some injuries benefit from icing 2–4 times a day. One exception is the immersion of the lower limbs in ice water for as much as 24 continuous hours to treat a horse at risk of laminitis. Refer to the section on laminitis (p. 136).

- Ice boots are an excellent investment, especially the kind with removable ice packs. As ice thaws in the inserts, exchange them for fresh frozen inserts to maintain a cold temperature.

- If ice boots aren't available, fill a sheath with ice water by using an inner tube or large empty intravenous fluid bag (available from your veterinarian) that extends from hoof or pastern to knee. Fill this sheath with crushed ice and water and secure it at the top of the cannon bone. Remain with the horse and monitor him while he is wearing this "sleeve."

- Commercial ice gel packs provide another option for icing. They can be thawed just enough to conform to the area needing cryotherapy. Secure a gel pack onto a leg with tape or a track bandage. This frees you up for other tasks—but stay with your horse to monitor him throughout the treatment. Replace the gel pack with a fresh one as it thaws.

- Frozen vegetables are also helpful for icing but thaw out very quickly; they need to be exchanged often to supply sufficient cold to an area. The advantage is they conform well to all crevices and irregularities on a limb.

STONE BRUISE OR FOOT ABSCESS

A stone bruise or thin soles can cause a horse to be lame, but not usually severely enough to have him refuse to put weight on the limb. A stone bruise benefits from hoof protection in a boot until it resolves.

There are times when a horse seems perfectly fine but when you look at him a few hours later, he is nearly non-weight-bearing lame on a leg. Among many possible reasons for this is the presence of a foot abscess.

How to Monitor for an Abscess

If there is no obvious injury to the hoof, push around on the heel bulbs and coronary band to check for tenderness or limb withdrawal. A foot abscess often tries to break out along the path of least resistance in these soft tissues; that area can be sore to touch and pressure or may show signs of wound drainage. Light rapping on the hoof wall with a hammer or a rock may cause the horse to pull the limb away if there is internal pressure and pain from an abscess. Some abscesses are too deep in the hoof to elicit a response on the

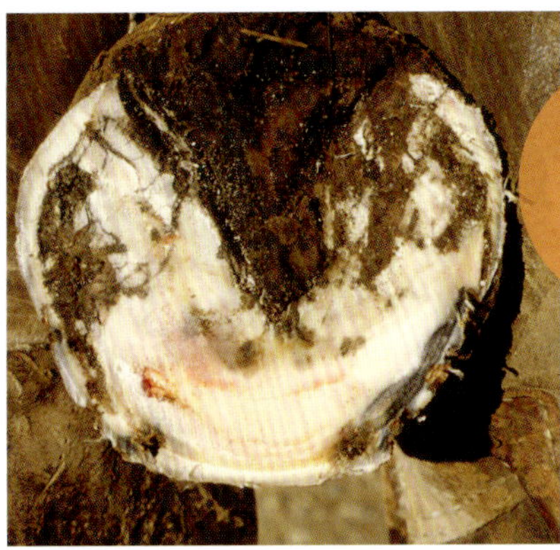

Bruising on the sole near the toe.

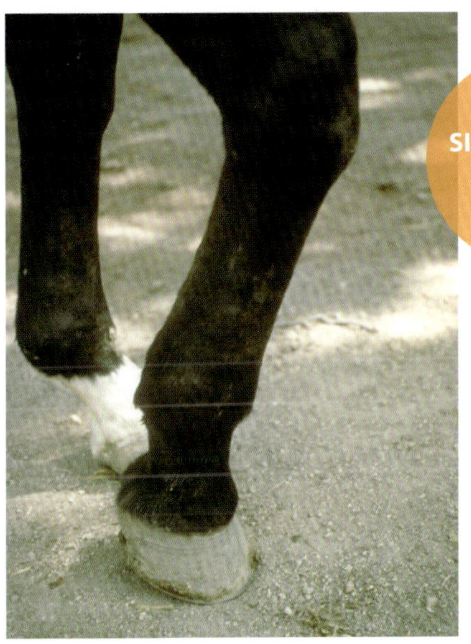

A foot abscess in the heel region causes a horse to raise his heel off the ground due to pain when standing or walking.

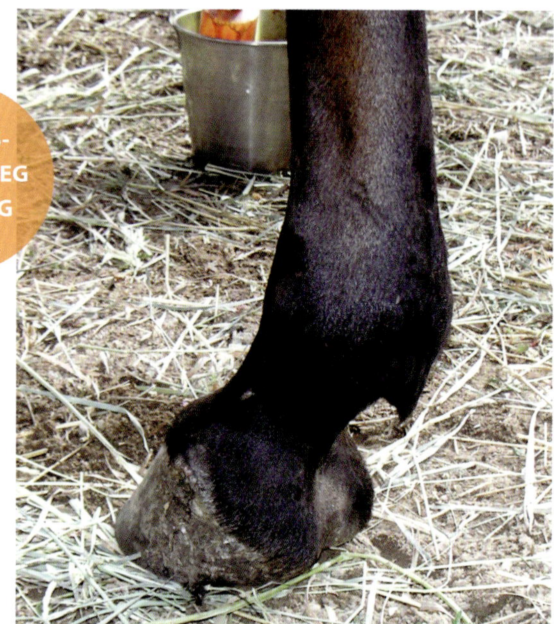

ABSCESS-RELATED LEG SWELLING

A foot abscess can cause swelling into the cannon area, as seen here. This can sometimes be confused with a tendon injury when in fact, the pressure from a foot abscess is what is causing swelling higher in the limb due to poor circulation.

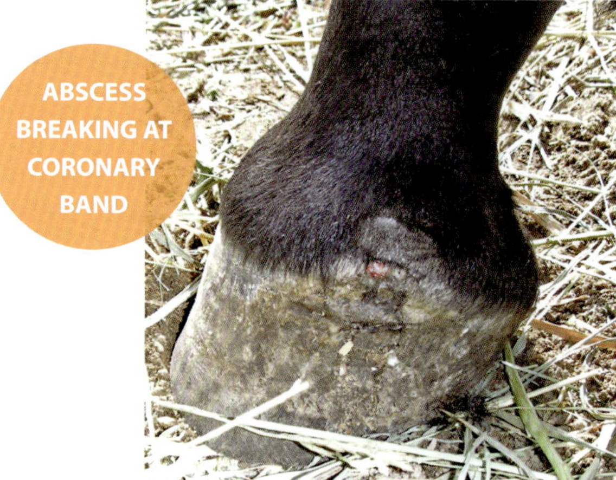

ABSCESS BREAKING AT CORONARY BAND

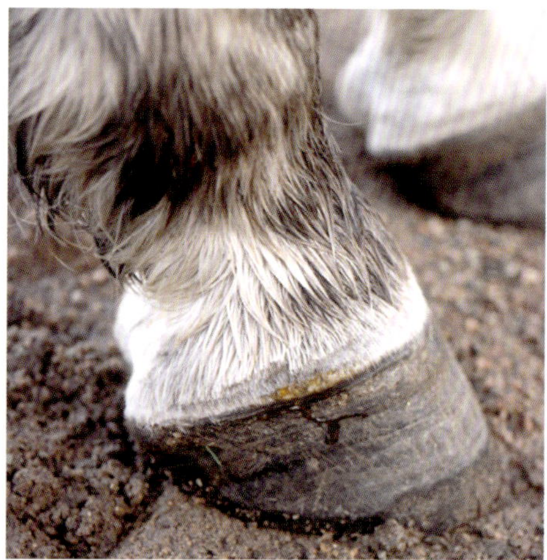

Since the hoof is a hard encasement, a foot abscess often breaks at the coronary band (shown here) or heel bulb, which are paths of least resistance through soft tissue.

external soft tissues, but the horse will likely react to pressure of hoof testers over the inflamed area of the sole.

At times, a hoof abscess is accompanied by swelling of the soft tissues that extend upward into the tendons along the back of the cannon bone; this may be confused with a tendon injury. Once the abscess breaks and drains, this swelling often resolves.

If it is obvious that your horse's problem is a stone bruise or a foot abscess, then proceed as described for a nail puncture (see next health issue) and use a synthetic boot to protect the horse's foot from further trauma.

NAIL PUNCTURE IN A HOOF

It is possible for a horse to step on a nail from a loose or twisted shoe—or just because there was a nail lying in his path. A puncture in the sole or at the angles of the bars generally heals uneventfully with appropriate care that includes opening the hole for drainage. But if the puncture is in the frog or the clefts of the frog, the horse needs immediate veterinary help without delay. If the nail has not yet penetrated deeply, rapid intervention prevents a nail from entering the navicular bursa or navicular bone, which could have life-threatening consequences.

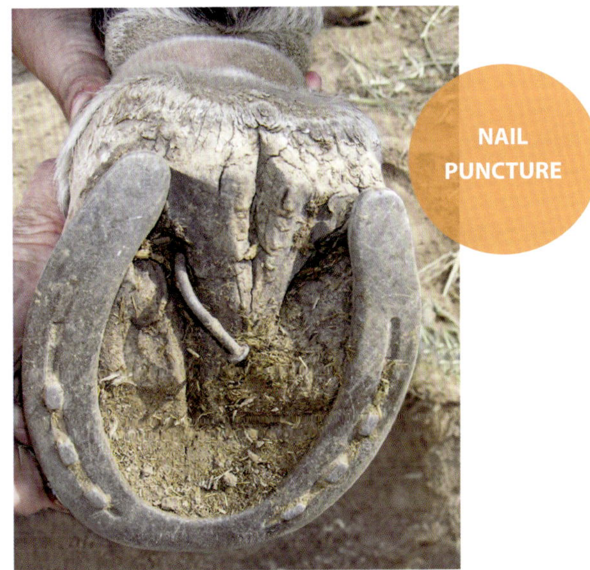

A nail puncture in the frog cleft is very serious because the nail is likely to have invaded the *navicular bursa*.

What to Do for a Nail Puncture in the Hoof

- Take photos of the embedded nail from the side and the bottom of the foot.

- Mark the location of the puncture with indelible ink (a Sharpie® pen), drawing a circle around it on the sole or frog.

- If there is danger of the horse putting weight on the foot and driving the nail deeper, pull it out after photographing it. Then mark the depth of penetration on the nail with an indelible pen. The part that entered the foot will be moist in appearance, whereas the portion of the nail that was not embedded in the foot will be dry; mark the place where the nail changes from moist to dry.

- Check if there is a soft or tender spot on the back of a heel bulb or along the coronary band where an abscess may be trying to drain. A horse may have stepped on a nail with infection underway but the nail did not remain in his foot. After a day or two, signs of infection may be obvious.

- Scrub the entire foot clean of debris, dirt, and manure.

- Soak the foot in a tub with warm water and dissolved Epsom salts, as much as will dissolve. Leave the foot in the soak bath for at least 15–20 minutes. Soak 2–3 times daily.

- Place the foot on a clean mat or towel and allow it to dry. Find an area free of debris in case the horse steps off the mat or towel so his foot remains clean.

- Squirt tamed povidone-iodine solution (Betadine) over the nail puncture, and apply Betadine-soaked gauze over the hole.

- Wrap the hoof in a bandage or place it in a synthetic protective boot. Refer to the section on bandaging (p. 105).

- Get veterinary attention as soon as possible so your vet can open the puncture and administer appropriate medical care for the location and depth of the nail puncture.

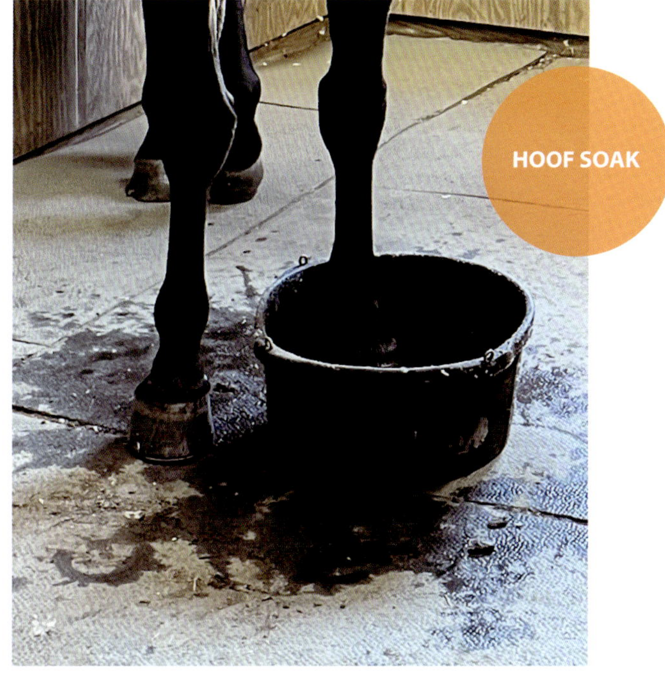

Soaking a hoof in warm water and Epsom salts.

HORSESHOE ISSUES

A problem with a horseshoe is a pretty common situation in the horse world.

- Your horse may have lost a shoe.

- The shoe may be loose, making a jingling sound with every footstep.

- The shoe may be sprung or twisted but is still attached to the hoof.

If the shoe is completely missing, protect the horse's hoof with a hoof boot.

If a shoe is just loose, hammer down the clinches to tighten them. Put something hard like a rock or hammer head behind the nail head on the bottom of the shoe, and then hammer directly over the nail clinches on the outside of the hoof. If the shoe doesn't seat down well with this method, pull it off altogether or place a hoof boot to keep it in place until a farrier is available.

A shoe may be sprung or twisted enough that the horse can't put his foot down comfortably while the shoe remains attached to the hoof. Pull the shoe off and put a boot on the foot until a farrier can come replace the shoe.

Pulling Off a Horseshoe

It is a good idea to know how to pull off a horseshoe, since a farrier or vet is not always available and you may not have a shoe-puller on hand.

- File away the nail clinches on the outside of the hoof until they are totally flush with the hoof wall. A multi-tool has a file that can do this.

- Hold the foot between your legs. Use pliers to pry the shoe off a little at a time, starting at each branch of the shoe and alternating from side to side. Rotate inward toward the frog as you pry it loose from heel to toe, not outward. Pulling outward is likely to pull off portions of the hoof wall. As you loosen the shoe, bang it back down periodically to expose the top of each horseshoe nail.

- Pluck out each loosened nail using pliers. This lets you remove the shoe easily without pulling off pieces of hoof wall and is less uncomfortable for a horse with a painful foot. The toe area is the last place to release.

■ Check for a nail that may have broken off in the hoof wall, and if there is one, try to pull it out. Usually a broken horseshoe nail embedded in the hoof won't cause much of a problem and you can leave it, but it could cause lameness if it sits too close to sensitive hoof tissue.

Is the Hoof Intact or Are Pieces Broken Off?

■ When a superficial piece of the outer hoof wall pulls off with the shoe, it isn't usually cause for alarm. This should grow out normally. However, if a large piece of hoof wall comes off, the hoof may need patching with epoxy until the wall toughens and grows down.

■ If the removed portion of the hoof wall involves deeper underlying dermis and subcutaneous tissue, then the wound has to heal by secondary intention (with granulation tissue) and needs wound care and bandaging. Refer to the section on wound care (p. 105).

Hot Nail

Most times, a farrier gets the job done correctly, but there are occasions where a horseshoe nail rests close to or within sensitive hoof tissue. The horse likely comes up acutely lame soon after. The best way to manage this is to pull out the problematic nail or remove the shoe altogether, as described on the previous page.

Once the nail or shoe is removed, drench the offending nail hole with antiseptic povidone-iodine solution, *not* tincture of iodine. It also helps to soak the foot in Epsom salt solutions once or twice a day for several days to help "draw" out any infection. Bandage the foot once it's dry:

■ Saturate gauze with povidone-iodine and place it over the nail opening.

■ Pack the foot in a hoof boot with a sheet of cotton covering the sole and up the sides to keep out dirt, gravel, or shavings.

■ Ensure that tetanus prophylaxis is up-to-date within the last eight months.

■ There should be no need for systemic antibiotics once the offending nail hole is open for drainage.

LAMINITIS

Inflammation within the hooves may start with the horse displaying subtle signs that develop into more obvious and significant pain. These include:

■ Lying down more often than usual or for long periods.

■ Decreased activity or disinterest in his surroundings (depression).

■ Shifting weight from limb to limb.

■ Pointing a throbbing foot.

■ Looking as though he is "walking on eggshells" or reluctant to move.

■ Difficulty turning.

■ A specific laminitis posture at a standstill: The horse rocks back on his hindquarters with his hind limbs far beneath his body (camped under), while both front legs are positioned well out in front of his body. This position relieves pressure on painful front toes.

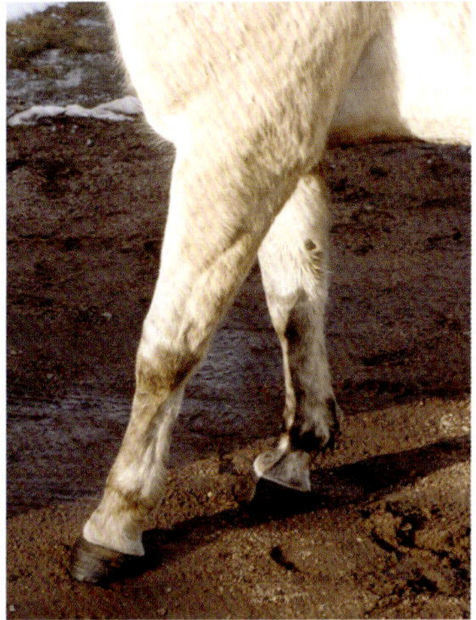

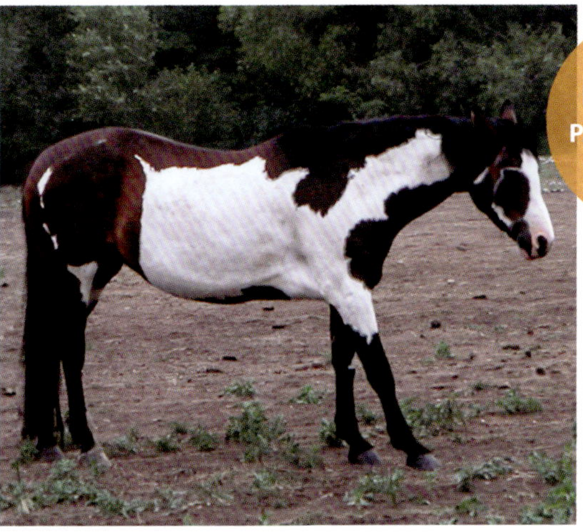

A horse often stands pointing a painful limb due to constant throbbing. In cases where both front or rear legs hurt, the horse is seen consistently shifting his weight from limb to limb.

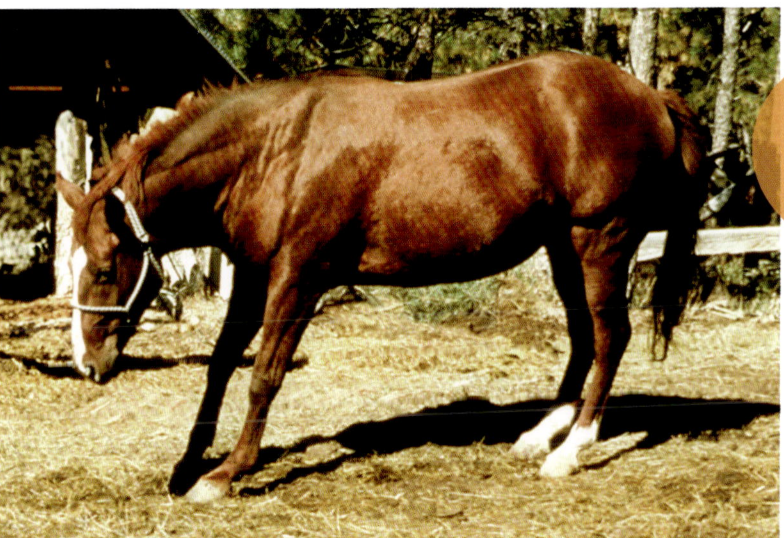

A severe laminitis posture has the horse with the front limbs placed way out in front, and rear limbs shifted under the body to try to get weight off painful front feet.

- His digital pulses (felt at the bottom edge behind the fetlocks—see photo on p. 27) are bounding.

The causes of laminitis are many, ranging from obesity and metabolic syndrome, endocrine changes including *pituitary pars intermedia dysfunction* (*PPID* or *Cushing's disease*), sepsis, and endotoxemia such as occurs with grain overload (see p. 61), uterine infection, retained placenta, enteritis, colitis, or other causes of intestinal dysfunction.

An episode of laminitis is a true emergency situation requiring prompt and immediate veterinary attention and aggressive therapy with anti-inflammatory medications and sole support.

What You Can Do in the Meantime

Place your horse's limbs in a deep bath of ice and water that covers the legs to the front knees. Include the rear legs to the hocks if it appears the horse is affected in all four limbs. Add ice as needed to keep the water chilled to 50 degrees Fahrenheit or just slightly colder. Consult with a veterinarian for how long the horse should be kept in this ice bath. Refer to the section on cryotherapy (p. 126).

- Administer NSAIDs as directed by a veterinarian.

- Provide sole support with deep sand, commercial frog pads specifically designed for this application, or builder's blue Styrofoam cut to fit the foot and bandaged in place with duct tape. Do *not* apply any tape or bandaging material on or over the coronary band. Be aware that foam or frog pads cannot be used if the horse is stabled in deep sand.

TENDON OR LIGAMENT INJURY—STRAIN OR SPRAIN

An athletic horse, or even one playing in a field, can injure a tendon or stretch a ligament that sprains a joint. At first, you may not see swelling. However, the horse may be quite lame and swelling usually develops soon after. What to look for:

- Check each leg and compare the injured leg to its opposite. Look for swelling or asymmetry.

- Run your hands down the back of the tendons. Gentle pressure can help you identify an area of discomfort. If a horse resents the squeeze on his tendons or suspensory ligaments, try the same analysis on the opposite leg and compare his responses. Not every reaction indicates true pain; some horses are simply sensitive to touch.

Once you find an area of concern:

- Ice is the best treatment for an acute injury. Apply ice boots or stand the horse in ice baths or a cold stream for 20–30 minutes to "cool down" the inflammatory response and provide pain relief. Intermittent icing periods over several days help curb the initial inflammation. Refer to the section on cryotherapy (p. 126).

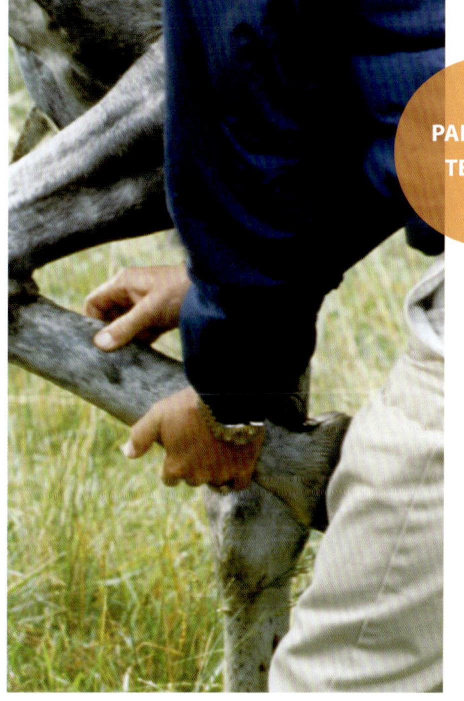

Palpating the superficial digital flexor tendon to identify an area of discomfort.

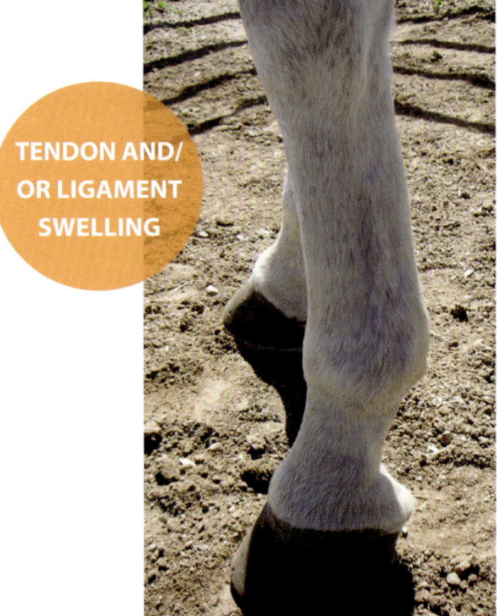
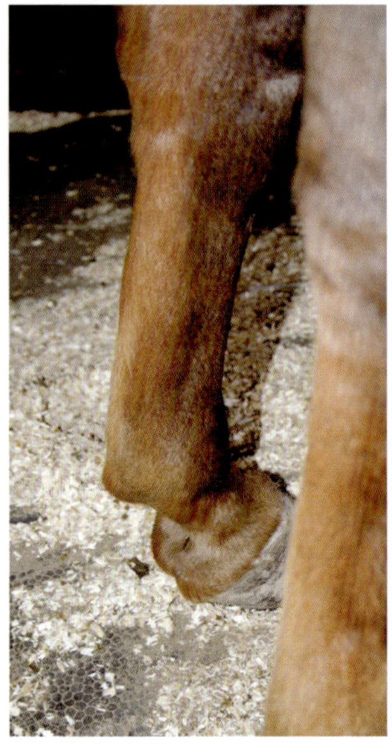
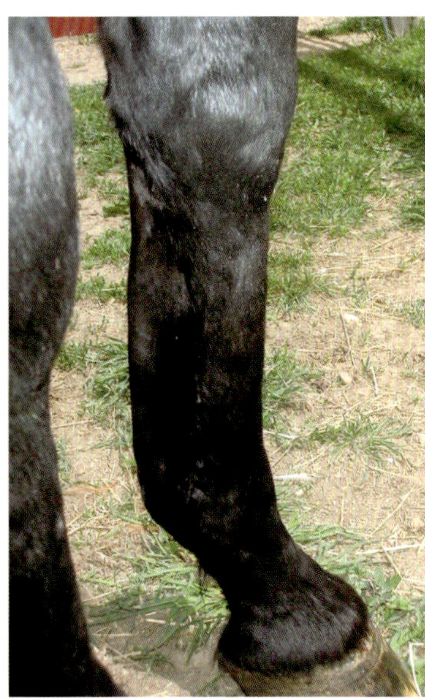

Swelling usually develops with a tendon or ligament injury.

- NSAIDs—phenylbutazone or flunixin meglumine (Banamine®) or firocoxib (Equioxx®)—are useful to curb inflammation. Use only under advisement by your veterinarian.

- A compression bandage keeps swelling in check. A standing wrap with many layers of cotton provides compression to minimize swelling, but even that many layers cannot "support" a tendon or ligament injury. Specialized medical boots with metal braces are necessary to take the load off a seriously injured tendon.

While a horse is recuperating from a tendon or ligament injury, confinement is important to allow healing and to prevent re-injury. The horse will need a sufficient period of rest and rehabilitation for his tissues to heal. Healing can be tracked well with ultrasound exams and veterinary consultation.

SERIOUS LIMB INJURY OR FRACTURE

A horse that is non-weight-bearing on a leg (Grade 5 lameness—see p. 120) may have incurred a fracture or suffered a torn tendon. This is a true emergency and you need professional help as soon as possible—but you can take steps to protect the horse from further damage until help can arrive.

The first step is to bandage the lower limb. Then add a splint to immobilize a possible fracture or tendon laceration. The joints above and below a fracture must be stabilized and immobilized. For example, a fracture of the front cannon bone requires bandaging from just above the hoof, or encompassing the hoof, to just below the elbow. For an injury in the pastern area, the entire foot, pastern, and fetlock need to be encased in bandaging and splinted.

- Bandage the area of injury by incorporating the joints above and below the fracture site or injury. Refer to the section on bandaging (p. 105).

- Pad the limb well by applying additional layers of cotton (1–2 rolls) or a pillow around the bandaged leg.

- To keep the padding in place, firmly wrap conforming roll gauze or self-adhesive elastic tape like VetWrap® or CoFlex around the limb. The extra padding not only holds bones or tendons in a fixed position but

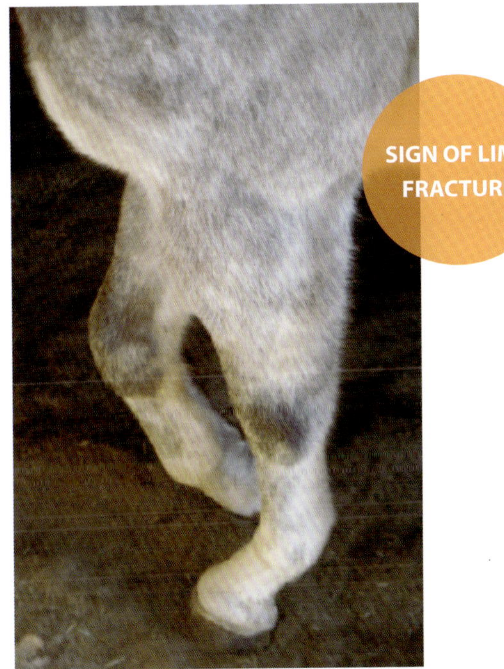

A non-weight-bearing limb fracture.

also limits the risk of compromising blood circulation from applying bandages too tightly. Stabilizing a fracture as much as you can also eases the horse's pain.

- Next, prepare to place a rigid, straight splint. Use 2-inch x 4-inch boards, broomsticks, or rake handles, or cut a piece of PVC pipe in half longitudinally to form two long semicircular pieces. Lay the two splint pieces along both sides (inside and outside—medially and laterally) of the leg. Extend the ends of the splint pieces to at least the bottom surface of the hoof, or slightly below. The tops of the splints must extend past the joint located above the fracture line.

- Secure the splints with self-adhesive bandaging.

- Confine the horse to a small area and keep someone with him at all times until veterinary help arrives, or until he can be transported (carefully) to a veterinary facility.

THE CAST OR TRAPPED HORSE

A horse confined to a stall or paddock may lie down and then become stuck in a corner or floor depression and be unable to rise because he can't get his hind legs beneath his body to push himself up. This is referred to as "being cast." This is an especially risky problem with big horses housed in small stalls or sheds, or if a horse falls down in a horse trailer.

In addition, an older horse with degenerative arthritis or another musculoskeletal disability, especially in his hind end, often has difficulty pushing himself off the ground with a sore leg. Despite no actual physical obstacle preventing him from rising, he is essentially cast.

A horse caught in a fence or entangled in wire is often unable to move. Some individuals wait quietly, while others thrash and create more damage.

How to Free a Cast Horse

The first thing to do is to remain calm. It's best to have another person or two to help when possible. People attempting to help a horse right himself should stay clear of flailing legs and head by approaching the horse from behind his withers. Ropes are useful to help flip the horse away from a wall, door, or fence.

- Always stay out of range of the arc of his legs and head when working to extricate the horse.

- Stay behind the horse by his withers, rather than in front of him by his head or chest.

It is important to move the cast horse as quickly as possible to prevent too much pressure from his body on his lungs and large muscle groups.

- Place a halter and lead rope on the horse to provide control of his head as you work, especially important once he starts to get to his feet.

- Loop a soft rope to each lower part of the front and hind legs closest to the ground, over each pastern.

- Encourage the horse to lie quietly while you do this.

- If the horse struggles while you are placing the halter and ropes, have someone kneel behind his neck; they should place a knee *firmly* on the horse's neck and pull his nose back toward their lap. This stops the horse from being able to try to rise, giving you time to loop the rope around his pasterns and begin to roll him over.

- You may be able to settle a struggling horse by placing a blindfold—a blanket or towel—so that it fully covers both of his eyes, to quiet him. Reassure and soothe the horse while placing the blindfold and ropes.

- Ensure your and others' personal safety by making sure there is a way out of the doorway, stall, or confined area you are working in if the horse struggles as he tries to get to his feet. Don't get yourself or others trapped!

- If you have assistance, pull together on the ropes around the horse's pasterns to roll him onto his other side, or to roll him out of his stuck position against a wall or fence or within a deep spot in a stall.

- Provided he is conscious, the horse will likely roll his head and neck on his own when you roll him over. It may not be necessary to guard his head unless there are obstacles his head could hit as he is rolled, or if he doesn't seem reasonably conscious or aware of his surroundings.

- Once his legs are all free, he should be able to get up on his own.

If a horse is trapped in an irrigation ditch, ravine, or other situation and must be moved a greater distance, never pull on or drag him by his limbs, tail, or head and neck. Use webbing (rather than rope) placed around his torso.

If the Horse Won't Rise Once Freed

If the horse won't or can't rise even after you've rolled him away from the physical obstacle that had trapped him, you will need additional people or horsepower to help get him to his feet:

■ While a horse attempts to rise, help him by lifting up on the base of his tail with your hands, as close as possible to where it attaches to his body. Pull straight up without bending the vertebrae at the base of the tail. Do not attempt this if you have back issues, and don't pull so hard that you risk back injury. It is best if there are 2–3 people helping lift the horse's hindquarters while another person stabilizes his head with the halter and lead rope.

■ The next step to try, if previous steps haven't helped the horse get to his feet, is to edge a strong strap or webbing beneath the horse's side just behind his front legs. Once it's in place, loop it around the girth area. Then, if feasible, lift the band with a tractor bucket to raise the horse to the point where he can find his legs and stand on his own.

■ If you lack a tractor or manpower and the horse still remains stuck on the ground but otherwise seems okay, then contact your local fire department. In many cases, those first responders are willing to come and help. They have plenty of equipment that can be used for this purpose but be sure to instruct them *not* to pull the horse by his legs, head, or tail. Leg ropes are only used to roll a horse over, not to lift him up. The safest way to lift a horse is with a strap looped around his girth area.

Entangled in Wire or a Fence

Fence boards and wire pose a hazard to curious horses that seek bits of grass or lie down for a good roll and then become entangled in the fence. A horse standing quietly is one that can probably be rescued as long as he continues to cooperate. Remember to stay calm and keep your body out of harm's way, especially if the horse decides to blow up as you attempt to free him. Try to stay on the other side of the fence from the horse and use wire cutters to cut wire away from an entrapped leg. Pay attention at all times to what the horse is doing and how he is reacting, and be prepared for a sudden eruption.

There are times when it is necessary to have veterinary assistance and sedation to safely free and move a horse caught in a fence. Don't proceed if a trapped horse is struggling or volatile. Wait for professional help. Offer hay to keep him quiet as long as possible while you await help.

Once the Horse Is on His Feet or Freed

Once a horse is no longer trapped or cast, check his vital signs and metabolic status, and look for any wounds that need attention. Refer to the sections on assessing vital signs (p. 26) and wound care (p. 97). Depending on how long a horse was trapped, he may need intravenous fluid support and treatment for wounds.

NEUROLOGIC ABNORMALITIES

A neurologic condition is a true emergency that not only poses a danger to the horse but also to humans. If this condition is caused by an infectious disease, that could also affect other horses in proximity to the sick horse.

Examples of clinical signs that indicate a neurologic issue:

- Lack of coordination and unsteadiness, referred to as *ataxia*.

- Stumbling.

- Loss of balance.

- Legs bumping each other (interference) when moving, or abnormal posture.

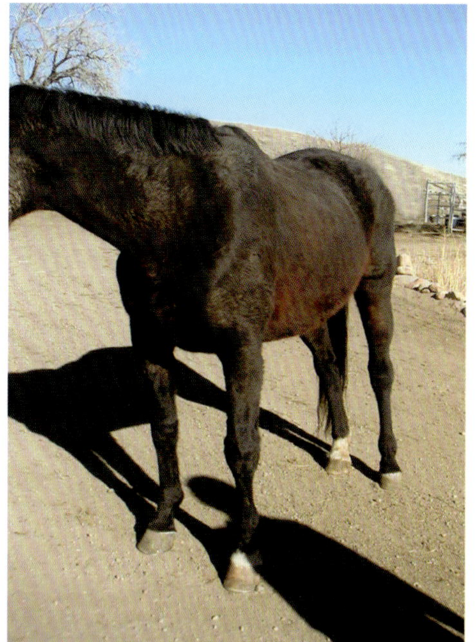
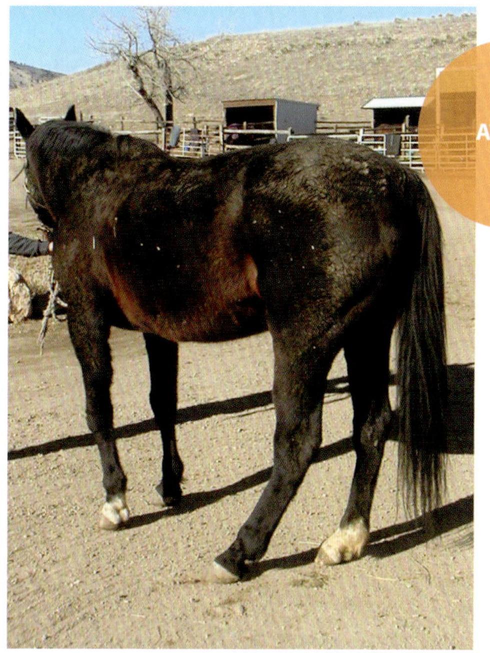

Ataxia of the rear limbs. Note that this horse's hind end is tilting to one side.

- Muscle weakness.

- Falling.

- Disinterest in surroundings, depression, or lower-than-normal activity level.

- Altered mental state—for example, a normally calm, happy horse begins to act anxious, volatile, or depressed.

- Lack of response to normal stimulation.

- Difficulty chewing or swallowing.

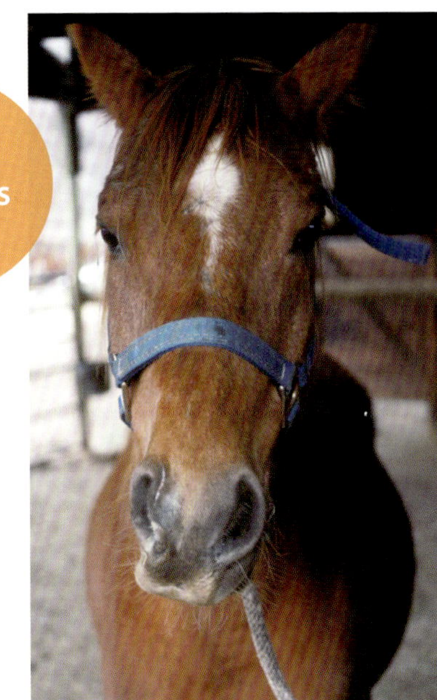

FACIAL PARALYSIS

Facial paralysis with muzzle pulled to one side.

- Drooping eyelid, lip, or ear.

- Muscle spasm.

- Urine dribbling, especially if the tail and buttocks seem limp or slack, or have poor muscle tone.

- Sudden blindness.

- Circling.

- Head pressing.

- Recumbent and unable to rise.

- Seizures.

- Some neurologic problems may mimic a lameness issue.

Neurologic Diseases That Require Emergency Attention

Infectious and Contagious Causes

- *Equine herpes myeloencephalopathy (EHM)* results from infection with *equine herpesvirus-1 (EHV-1)*, which is a respiratory virus that is highly transmissible between horses.

- Rabies is a serious and potentially fatal neurologic disease that is also able to infect humans and other animals. Initial signs of rabies are non-specific. The horse may simply just seem lame or "not right"; this progressively turns into more obvious signs of rabies with behavioral and neurologic signs.

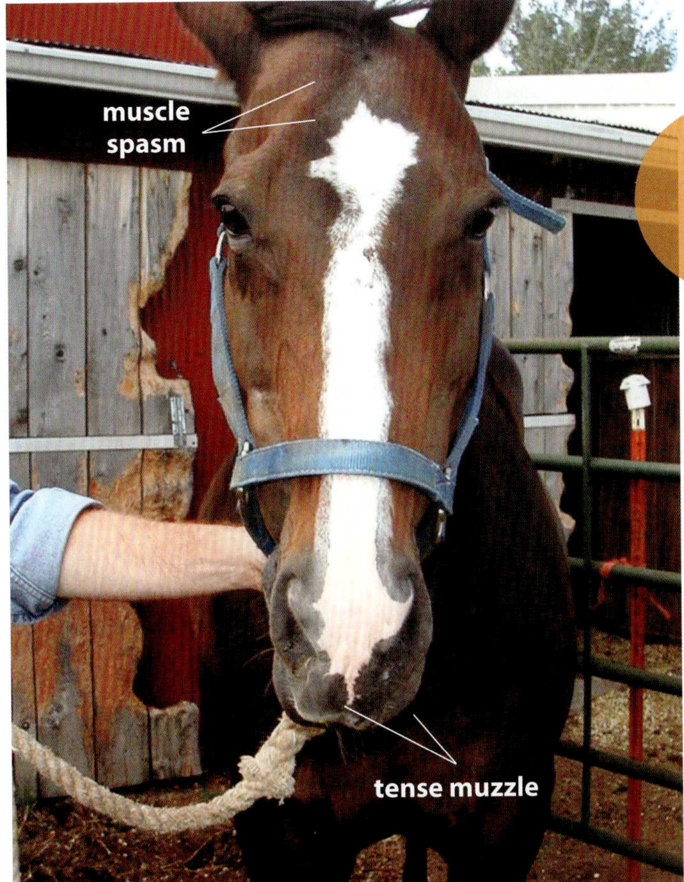

An example of West Nile virus cranial nerve abnormalities: muscle spasm of the forehead and tense muzzle.

Non-Contagious Causes

- *West Nile virus* and *Eastern* or *Western equine encephalitis virus*, all of which are transmitted by mosquitoes to horses, not from horse to horse.

- *Equine protozoal myeloencephalitis (EPM)* affects the spinal cord and cranial nerves; horses become infected by consuming—in feed or water—contaminated feces from opossums or other animals.

■ *Anaplasmosis*, caused by tick bites, may elicit rare neurologic problems. Refer to the section on fever (p. 64).

■ *Tetanus* creates odd neurologic abnormalities that mimic other neurologic or musculoskeletal signs: stiffness; displacement of the third eyelid to at least partially cover the globe of the eye; muscle spasms; and lockjaw that makes it difficult for the horse to open his mouth.

■ *Lyme disease*, caused by bites of ticks infected with *Borrelia burgdorferi* bacteria, can create neurologic signs, including depression, low

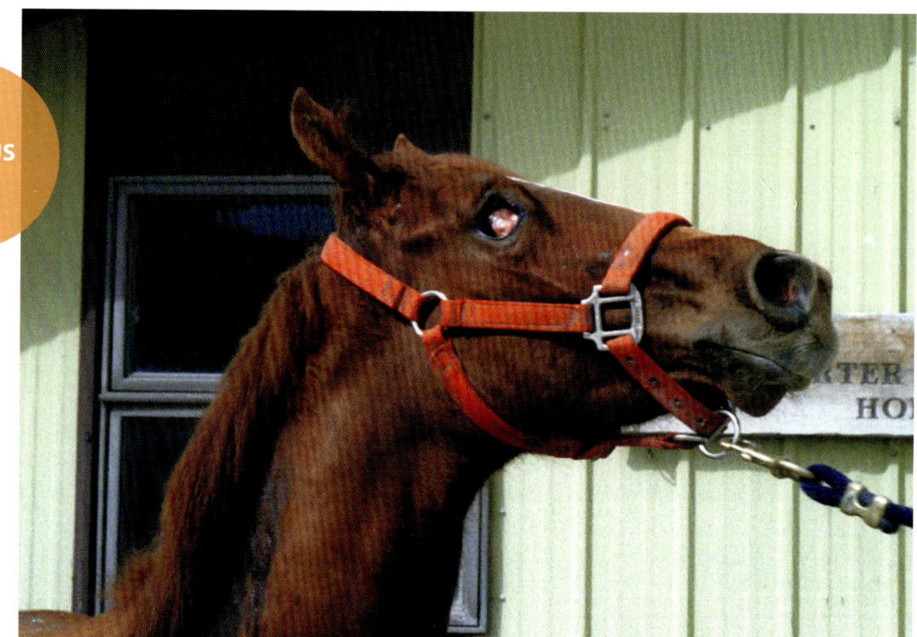

Stiff and rigid musculature and limbs, open nares (nose openings locked in position), and third eyelid prolapse are typical signs of tetanus.

activity and disinterest in surroundings, skin hypersensitivity, ataxia, head tilt, and brain inflammation (p. 64).

- *Botulism* results from ingestion of or contamination of a wound with spores of a specific bacteria, *Clostridium botulinum*. An affected horse shows *flaccid paralysis*—he cannot tense his muscles so they are slack without tone.

- Moldy corn poisoning.

- A middle or inner ear infection that is often associated with a head tilt and/or ataxia (incoordination).

West Nile virus, equine encephalitis virus, EPM, botulism, Lyme disease, Anaplasmosis, moldy corn poisoning, ear infections, and tetanus are ***not*** transmissible directly between horses. Other horses near a sick horse may also be affected by these conditions most likely because they share the same environment as the sick horse and have been exposed to the same contaminants, neurotoxins, or insects rather than because they caught it from the sick horse.

What to Do for a Neurologic Emergency

- Contact a veterinarian immediately.

- Assume a horse may have rabies until it is confirmed otherwise. If a horse has not been well immunized against rabies (or even if he has been immunized), use all personal protection equipment options available to you to protect you from potential contact with a horse's saliva or mucous membranes. Handle the horse as little as possible and await professional care.

■ If a horse demonstrates any neurologic clinical signs or may have been exposed to a contagious infectious disease like herpesvirus or rabies, ***isolate him immediately***, away from other horses. In the case of rabies, as few people as possible should interact with the horse and only when wearing personal protective equipment.

■ Place the horse in a spacious and well-bedded stall. Refer to the section on biosecurity recommendations (p. 154).

■ Provide easily accessible food and water. If you think the horse might have botulism, inspect all food for possible contaminants, and use a different source of feed from what he had been fed.

■ As few people as possible should handle a horse with a neurologic issue, and they should only do so in a spacious area to avoid injury. Ensure you are able to stay out of the way of an ataxic or unstable horse that might fall.

PART 3

PREPARING FOR GENERAL EMERGENCIES

BIOSECURITY RECOMMENDATIONS

Biosecurity is a word that describes a system of management protocols that limit transmission and spread of infectious diseases like bacteria, viruses, or fungal infections wherever horses congregate. A horse—whether he is a carrier or incubating an illness—does not necessarily show obvious signs of sickness but may still infect other horses. It's important to follow these procedures even when no horses on a farm or at a venue appear ill.

Practical biosecurity strategies are important, particularly in the face of a potential infectious disease outbreak if there is even a single case of confirmed illness on the property.

- Keep tabs on every horse on the property and monitor them for any abnormal signs.

- Know what is normal for each individual horse and have barn personnel communicate if anything is amiss with a horse's attitude, appetite, or manure and urine output.

- Any time something seems out of the ordinary, take the horse's rectal temperature. It is also important to monitor rectal temperature twice a day on any new horses to the property. This precaution is done for up to 14 days. Temperatures exceeding 101 degrees Fahrenheit in a horse that isn't feeling himself is a good reason to isolate the horse and implement biosecurity precautions. Refer to the sections on assessing vital signs (p. 26) and rectal temperature (p. 38).

Isolation Procedures

Isolating a sick horse quickly can mean the difference between one case of illness and a full-blown outbreak on a farm. Until a veterinarian can come to determine the cause of the illness, you can take steps to contain an outbreak.

- Set up an isolation area a good distance away from other horses. A minimum distance for controlling spread of a disease like *equine herpesvirus* is at least 10 yards (30 feet); diseases like *equine infectious anemia (EIA)* or *piroplasmosis* require 200 yards (600 feet) between infected horses and other equids.

- Post clear signs to warn people about the location of the isolation area and the seriousness of maintaining that isolation.

Isolation isn't just about distance. It is also about committing to implementation of multiple biosecurity practices.

- Disinfect footwear before entering or leaving the isolation area, using bactericidal and virucidal footbaths or mats.

- There should be ***no*** opportunity for nose-to-nose contact or shared water between a sick horse and other horses. This also applies to new horses on the property that should have no such contact with resident horses during a quarantine period.

- Do all feeding and cleaning chores for a sick horse in the isolation area only *after* taking care of other non-exposed horses.

- Don't allow watering hoses to touch containers or the water within the containers.

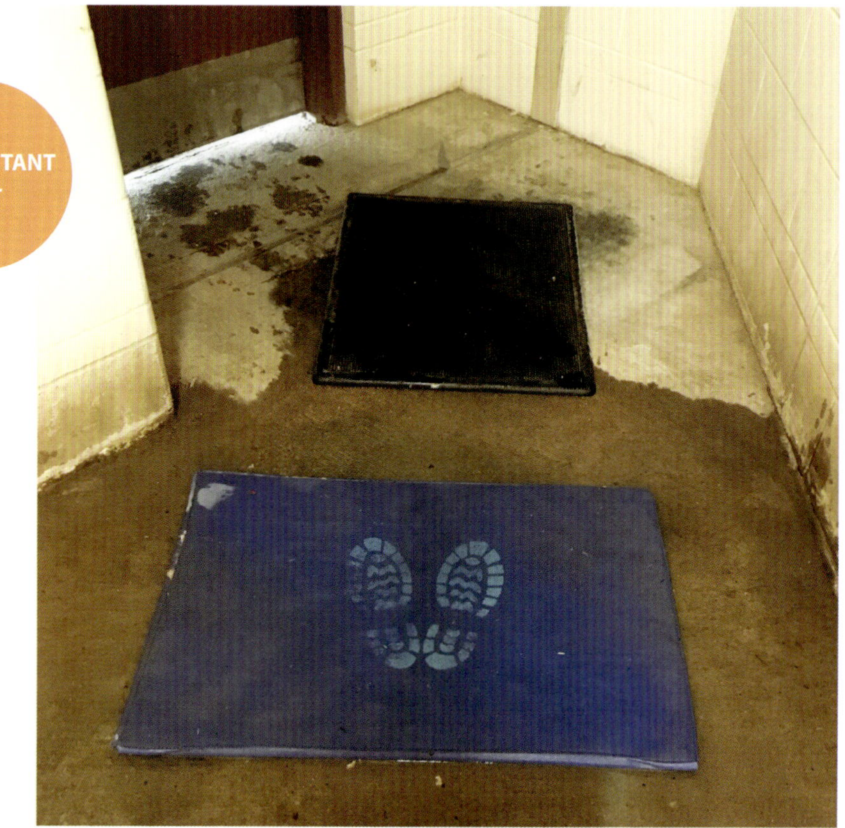

A disinfectant mat (shown here) is one method of disinfecting footwear; a better option is to use antiseptic footbaths.

- Keep separate equipment like manure buckets, rakes, wheelbarrows, tractors, blankets, grooming tools, and tack for the isolation area; don't use the same set of tools for the sick horse and for other horses.

- Use one set of shovels, rakes, and pitchforks for manure cleanup, and one set for moving and spreading out fresh bedding—never use the same tools for both jobs.

- Label the tools and implements used in an isolation area so they aren't inadvertently mixed in with equipment used around other horses.

- Color code buckets to make it clear what is used where; you might decide to use red buckets only in your highest-risk isolation area, for example.

- Disinfect the wheels, tires, and external parts of tractors, wheelbarrows, and manure spreaders. Use disinfectants such as Chlorox® (¼ cup per gallon of water), VirKon® S, Tek-trol®, or One Stroke Environ® solutions.

- Carefully dispose of contaminated cleaning solutions and bedding in a transport system that is used only for this purpose.

- Think about the direction of water drainage; make sure there is no chance of water from the isolation area draining into a space with other horses, or vice versa.

- Manage manure storage and eliminate standing water to minimize flies and mosquitoes, which can carry disease between horses that are physically separated from each other.

- Be aware that children and small animals (cats and dogs, and domestic fowl) as well as wild animals (rodents, raccoons, and opossums, for example) can carry disease around a farm. The movements of cats, dogs, chickens, and children are manageable to some extent but those of wild animals are not.

- Remove anything that might attract wild animals to the areas where horses are kept, and store feed supplies in closed rooms or buildings, using animal-proof containers made of metal or heavy plastic and secured with lids. Clean up spilled or leftover feed and remove trash regularly.

- Wash your hands with liquid soap in between handling different horses—a simple hygiene practice for everyone to follow. A general rule is to sing "Happy Birthday" twice while scrubbing, to make sure you're washing long enough for it to be effective. Hand sanitizers with a minimum of 61 percent alcohol can be used if hand washing isn't an option and there is only minimal contamination on your hands. Apply an appropriate amount (a blob of 2–3 centimeters diameter—about an inch) of hand-sanitizing gel, rub it in well, and then allow it to dry for 15–20 seconds.

- Observe a sick horse closely and keep a daily log of his rectal temperature, attitude, appetite, and manure and urine output. Know the normal vital signs for an individual horse so there is immediate and early recognition that a horse "isn't quite right." (Refer to the section on assessing vital signs on p. 26.) Follow up on any signs of malaise, fever, diarrhea, cough, ocular or nasal discharge, or neurologic issues.

DISASTER PREPAREDNESS

As natural disasters become more prevalent with climate change even in areas where they are least expected, it is a good idea to map out a plan, just in case. The American Association of Equine Practitioners (AAEP) proposes specific helpful recommendations to heed for an impending natural disaster. Let's look at some strategies to help you respond and protect your horses in such a situation.

Put a Plan in Place

- Make a plan and put it in writing.

- Post it in multiple areas—barn entrances, tack room, horse trailer—preferably in a laminated or waterproof casing.

- Email it to yourself for easy access on your phone, and to other horse owners in your barn.

- If in a multi-owner barn, practice the plan in advance of an emergency situation to identify protocols that need fine-tuning.

- Ensure that all horses are trained to load into a trailer at a moment's notice.

- Include an emergency kit, important equine medications, and each horse's medical information when possible.

- Remember that human evacuation takes precedence if there is limited time.

- Keep yourself, friends, and family safe.

Truck and Trailer Preparation

- Ensure that your truck and trailer are in working condition and ready to go.

- During seasons of concern, make sure your gas/diesel tank is full.

- Plan ahead for other contacts who can help haul your horses if you are not able to or are not present at the time of the crisis.

- Put in the truck addresses and directions to locations that accept horses during an evacuation event so you know where to go.

- Have on board plenty of hay and water to accommodate your horses for a couple of days.

When to Evacuate

- If there is ample notice—hurricanes or potential flooding—leave at least 72 hours in advance of the crisis.

- Remember that if everyone leaves at once close to an event, then there may be road closures or difficulty negotiating traffic.

- Plan for at least two possible evacuation routes in case of road closures or traffic.

What to Do If You Choose Not to Evacuate or Are Unable to Evacuate Your Horses

- If you don't plan on evacuating or are unable to get your horses out, ensure that there is ample food, water, and necessary supplies available for at least 3-4 days for the horses and other pets remaining on the property.

- Fill plastic barrels with ample water in advance because if electricity goes out, it may be impossible to pump water. It is also possible that well water may become contaminated following a natural disaster—it is best to have plenty of safe drinking water on hand.

■ Label each horse with your phone number, using livestock crayon on the rump or neck, or use a Sharpie® pen on the hooves.

■ Cattle tags can be braided into the horse's mane and marked with specific information.

■ Use a breakaway or leather halter with contact info on it. Do not use synthetic halters.

■ A fly mask may help protect eyes from flying debris.

■ Ensure that any objects that can become airborne—tools, buckets, wheelbarrows, arena equipment—are secured and put away.

■ Don't turn horses loose into areas with which they are unfamiliar. It is better to leave them in a fenced pasture that is free of farm equipment or other debris. That also keeps them off the roads or footpaths where they may be invisible in the dark.

■ Put compatible horses together when possible.

■ It is not necessarily safe to leave a horse in a barn as he could become trapped or severe winds can wreak havoc on a structure, with flying debris or destruction.

■ In the event of wildfire, leave horses in pasture away from combustible buildings, hay, or equipment.

■ Safely store ample fuel for a generator if you have one, and know the correct way to use it.

Documents to Have on Hand

- Have each horse's documents in a secure folder to go with or stay with each horse:

  - Health records.

  - Vaccination history.

  - Current Coggins test.

  - Medications (dose and frequency) that each horse receives, labeled with horse's name.

  - Horse photos for later identification if necessary.

  - Microchip information if a horse is microchipped.

  - Horse insurance information and documentation with contacts to call.

  - Medical directives for each horse—this is important in case a horse needs medical care and you are not available to communicate what you will authorize.

  - Emergency contact list of people who are authorized to make decisions about a horse's care on your behalf.

  - Contact information for your veterinarian, and an alternative backup veterinarian.

  - Contact information for local fire, police, and other first responders.

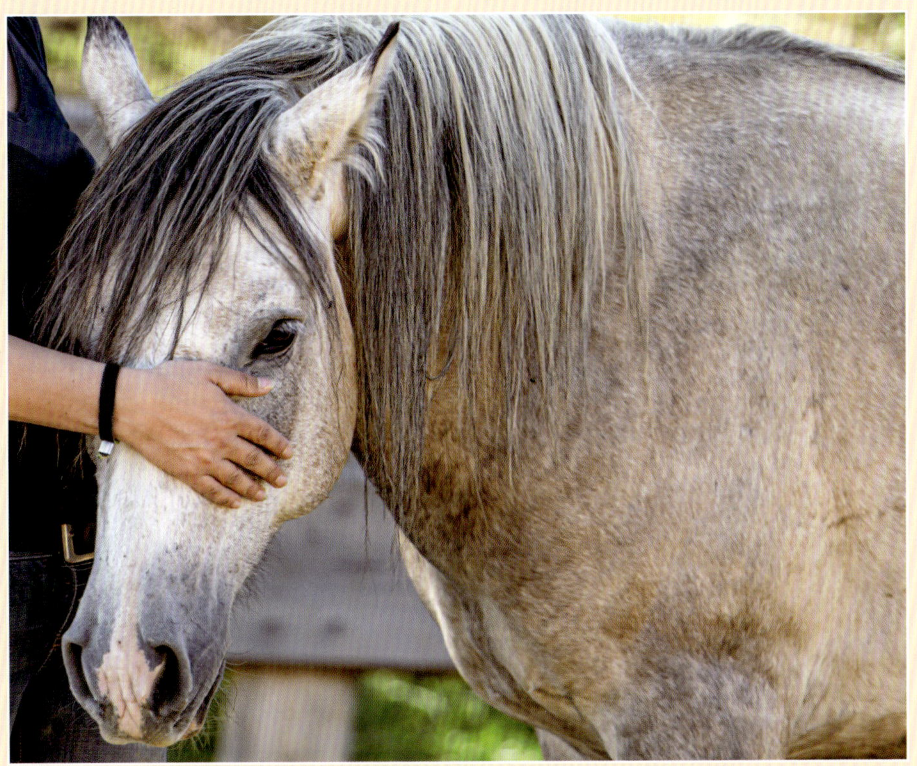

EMERGENCY TAKEAWAYS

In these pages, I have provided common equine emergency situations and basic tools to care for your horse until your veterinarian arrives. The objective is to help ensure a positive result once professional attention is administered, while keeping you and your horse as safe as possible. Every equine emergency is different. Consider the situation in context of urgency and seriousness when determining what steps are most critical and what to do first.

Guidelines for a
POSSIBLE EMERGENCY

General guidelines are helpful in a crisis. Remember the following points when dealing with an emergency:

- Your safety is paramount. You cannot help your horse if you are dealing with your own injury. If your well-being is jeopardized because your horse won't tolerate your help, then wait for professional assistance.

- Try to get a general sense of the health issue or injury—behavior that seems to indicate illness or location and extent of a wound, as examples. With information in hand, call your veterinarian to request assistance. Communicate what you have observed and when you first observed it, and your location. Ask for a likely arrival time and discuss steps your veterinarian would like you to take in the interim.

- Once the veterinary professional has been alerted to the emergency, follow your veterinarian's outlined steps if provided, or proceed with suggested steps in this book to secure, stabilize, and prepare your horse for veterinary care.

- Throughout, remain as steady and focused in your movements and actions as possible. Horses are sensitive to human emotions. By remaining calm, it is more likely that your horse will also stay calm.

INDEX